Healing through Touch

A History and a Review
of the Physiological Evidence

John T. Cottingham

Rolf Institute
Boulder, Colorado

ACKNOWLEDGMENTS

There are many people who have provided information, encouragement, criticism, and direction in the writing of this book. I would like to express my deepest appreciation to the following: Jim Asher, Bob Brown, Sue Carter-Porges, Joanne Huff, Emmett Hutchins, Peter Levine, Peter Melchior, Stacey Mills, Joan Murray, George Ordal, Jim Oschman, Stephen Porges, James Weyhenmeyer, Heather Wing, Tom Wing, and Carl Woese.

I am also grateful to my clients for sharing their experiences and ideas concerning somato-therapy.

A special thanks to Neal Powers and Richard Stenstadvold and the Rolf Institute for their support in publishing the book.

My deep appreciation to Sue Tristano for her masterful job of editing the final version.

Finally, my thanks to my wife, Mary Rose, whose commitment, patience, and love in editing the many early drafts of this manuscript made it all possible.

FOREWORD

The number of books published each year on any subject is enough to stagger even the most vivid imagination. It is then a bold undertaking to recommend yet another book to a world which is rapidly running out of trees from which to make the paper.

This volume, however, is one which I am convinced merits attention. I recommend it on the grounds that it is unusually valuable in at least two respects. First, it is an excellent work of history, written from a point of view rarely found in the familiar literature pertaining to the somatic arts and sciences. Its second quality, which makes it particularly worthwhile, is its survey of the scientific investigations into the "mechanisms" which underlie these somatic approaches and how this experimental evidence supports their therapeutic uses.

The term **somatic** (from the Greek, meaning "bodily") is used to describe a wide range of techniques which are included in this book. (It is used by Thomas Hanna, who edits and publishes a fine journal called *Somatics*.) It expresses the intention held in common by the creators of these systems: to restore the unity of body and mind to our considerations of the human organism.

The choice of someone to write a foreword was accomplished through the use of a relatively simple set of criteria: I liked the book. John Cottingham liked that. Since I feel that the book speaks pretty well for itself, it is probably best that I state plainly and briefly just what it is I liked about it.

In writing this book, Cottingham has done a great service for practitioners, teachers, researchers, and writers in these therapeutic disciplines; but the best part is that it is written in such a way that it is easily understandable to anyone who may have an interest in the subject.

Most of the written material tends to take the form either of books and papers by the pioneers who have devised various somatic systems, or by others attempting to explain the original work, or to expand upon the theme. In both cases, the context may be a narrow one designed to refer only to a particular mode of somatic technique—the ideas of one school of thought. Relatively little has been available which seeks to explore the interrelationships that connect the thought and activity of these innovators, as well as the thing-in-itself. For example, first there are writings by Andrew Still, Moshe Feldenkrais, F.M. Alexander, and Ida Rolf. In the next category are the works of William Sutherland, Yochanan Rywerant, Frank Pierce Jones, and Don Johnson—their students. Finally, this is followed by the efforts of such people as John Lilly, Charles Dart, and John Dewey, who have reaped benefit from the work of these authors. It is left to the present volume to begin an exploration which attempts to discover the common ground from which these systems take their substance.

The author chose a difficult path to follow: writing one book from two different perspectives. Since he is involved personally in both practice and research, it may be assumed that he knows what he is talking about. Often, however, this closeness to the subject carries some disadvantage for a writer, as well as the obvious advantages. From such a perspective, one may be in a position to perceive an enormous amount of detail, yet be deprived of a view of the whole field. Cottingham seems to have circumvented this perceptual cul-de-sac and to have arrived at a vantage point which is far enough removed from his chosen subject that it affords a large view, yet close enough so that the details are not obscured.

Any worker in this field who entertains an urge to write further on the subject now has a steady tree, rooted deeply in good soil, from which to observe the landscape. It is possible to begin from a rich and long tradition which has been, until now, partially hidden from view. We are left with a good historical document, as well as a clear and accurate presentation of some of the fascinating stories beginning to unfold from the work of scientific investigators.

The various somatic approaches represented here were brought into being by people possessed of enormous curiosity. They were gifted and persistent investigators, who spent most of their lives wrestling with the problems of life, asking hard questions in an attempt to separate essential and significant information from what is merely accidental. They attempted to uncover, in each case, a true theme which might grow into a unified work of art, even in the face of the small likelihood that this fruition would be realized within their own lifetimes.

Although the pioneers whom I have personally known were confronted with often contradictory notions about the world around them and the place of humankind in it, they shared one common notion—that they were part of the long story of human enquiry, connected to those who went before and to those who were to come after them. We who are their effective heirs need reminding from time to time of the larger context in which we live and work. It is far too common an error to believe that the particular set of ideas one has espoused (and occasionally seeks to own or to hold a mortgage upon) has sprung suddenly up, as if by magic, from virgin soil. In giving us this book, John Cottingham has helped to set the record straight—not only for those of us who work in the "bodily arts and sciences," but also for the people who benefit from the services of practitioners in the somatic arts.

Ida Rolf remarked that the people she selected to educate as practitioners of her work, often chosen partly because of a demonstrated ability to write, became so involved in practice that they never wrote another word! As sincerely and thoroughly as she disliked being proven wrong, I believe that she would have been delighted with this book.

Peter Melchior, Rolfing Instructor
February 1986
Lyons, Colorado

PREFACE

Healing through touch goes back further than the 5,000 years of recorded history; prehistoric cave paintings portray the "laying on of hands" for the sick and injured.

This book has developed over the last 15 years and originated from my growing interest in the somato-therapies (somato, the Greek word for "body"). It is a personal journey that led me to experience most of the therapies described in the following pages. Some of the methods, particularly the Rolfing technique, affected my physical being or "core" in a very literal sense as well as opening emotional-psychological dimensions.

This exploration has been personally eventful in many ways: a three-month experience in an ashram; a frustrating year and a half in medical school; training in body therapies; and most recently as an investigator of somato-techniques and the autonomic nervous system.

The book is intended both for the curious reader and the serious student/practitioner who longs to know more about the historical background of these methods as well as the physiological basis of their therapeutic effectiveness.

Its purpose is twofold. Part I reviews the systems of somato-therapy from a historical perspective. Emphasis is placed on: (1) the cultural and philosophical orientations from which the techniques developed, and (2) how most modern somato-procedures have borrowed and "rediscovered" methods from the earlier ancient systems. The goal, then, of Part I is a descriptive one, serving the purpose of a "field study," providing the reader with a cultural context for healing techniques that have existed since the beginnings of written history.

Part II, in contrast, examines the scientific literature concerning somato-techniques and their effects on various physiological systems: circulatory, connective tissue, nervous, neuromuscular, autonomic, and the endogenous opiate peptides. A chapter is devoted to each of these systems, and possible mechanisms and theories are discussed. Therapeutic benefits, both known and potential, are examined in light of the physiological evidence presented.

Part II assumes that the reader has a basic knowledge of human physiology and anatomy. However, overviews are provided in each chapter to introduce terms and concepts.

I trust that the reader's exploration of healing through touch will be as rewarding and fruitful as my own.

John T. Cottingham
Champaign, Illinois
March, 1986

CONTENTS

Part I — Historical Perspective

Part II — Physiological Evidence

PART I
HISTORICAL PERSPECTIVE

Tao produced the One.
The One produced the two.
The two produced the three.
And the three produced the ten
thousand things.
The ten thousand things carry the **yin**
and embrace **yang** and through
the blending of the **qi** they
achieve harmony.

—*Lao Tzu*

CHAPTER 1
ANCIENT CHINESE MEDICINE AND ACUPUNCTURE

One of the earliest forms of somato- or "body" therapy originates from the ancient civilization of China some 5,000 years ago. To appreciate the theory and technique of acupuncture, classical Chinese philosophy must first be examined since Chinese medicine grew out of this world view.

Man was seen as a reflection of the larger universe, a microcosm within a macrocosm. Both were subject to the universal natural law or underlying reality, called the **Tao** (Watts, 1957).

Around 3,000 BC, legend has it that the first of three great Chinese emperors, **Fu Hsi,** put forth the Tao concept in terms of two complementary primordial principles of the natural world: **yin** and **yang.** Yin was expressed as the feminine, soft, intuitive, nurturing, and receptive force. Yang was considered the masculine, light, firm, rational, arousing, and assertive force (Kaptchuk, 1983).

Although the Taoist philosophy may sound to the modern reader chauvinistic, nothing superior is implied in the yang principle to the yin. In fact they can exist only in relation to one another; every human being — as well as the rest of nature — having varying degrees of both elements (Lao Tzu, 1972). Instead of viewing yin and yang as two separate, discrete forces, traditional Chinese thought describes them as two undulating poles of a single pattern:

1

> The universe is said to be in a state of constant cyclic motion, fluctuating between the two complementary forces of Yin and Yang. The human body is also viewed as being in a state of constant cyclic motion, pulsating rhythmically between Yin and Yang influences, seeking perfect balance . . . (Chu, Yeh, and Wood, 1979, p. 5).

About 200 AD the dialogues of the third great emperor, **Shen Nung,** (accession 2,697 BC) were collected into the Chinese medical classic, *Nei Jing (The Yellow Emperor's Classic on Internal Medicine)* (Veith, 1972). It was here that the technique of acupuncture is first described in detail.

The practice of acupuncture involved the stimulation of specific points along the body, usually by the insertion of tiny, solid needles; but massage and other forms of pressure were also used.

The prehistoric forerunner of the acupuncture needle is probably found in the flint needles of Neolithic man (5,000-7,000 BC) which were inserted into the skin for the relief of pain and sickness. Such practices were also found in traditional Eskimo and African medicine, where sharp stones were used to scratch the skin's surface (Stanway, 1979).

According to traditional acupuncture theory, disease appears when the balance between the primordial forces of yin and yang is lost. The imbalance may be due to poor diet, trauma, stress, etc. In turn, the expression of disease is evident along specific acupuncture points located on or just below the skin's surface; those loci become tender to the touch, swollen or discolored (Mann, 1973).

The actual movement of the yin and yang forces through the body is called the movement of **qi**, translated literally as "air" or "breath" but better understood in English as "life force" or "vital energy" (Chu, Yeh, and Wood, 1979).

The qi circulates through the body by means of 14 channels or pathways called **meridians.** In classical acupuncture, there are 360 pressure points on these meridians. The meridians are classified in terms of yin-yang attributes as are the individual points. The flow of qi is carried through the body from one meridian to the next in an endless sequence of meridian cycles (Mann, 1973).

Of the 14 meridians, 12 are double meridians associated with the 12 internal organs conceptualized in Chinese medicine — each meridian pair located symmetrically, one on each side of the body.

Six "hollow" organs, considered yang in quality, are involved in "secretion" (large intestine, stomach, small intestine, bladder, gall bladder, and triple-warmer). Six "solid" organs are described as yin and function in "storage and collection" (lung, spleen, heart, kidney, liver, and circulation-sex). The "triple-warmer" and "circulation-sex" meridians have no correlate in Western anatomy. However, the circulation-sex appears functionally related to the endocrine system; and the triple-warmer meridian seems involved in the "heat" or metabolism of the respiratory, digestive, and reproductive systems (Bresler, 1981). (See Table 1.)

YIN	YANG
Lung	Large Intestine
Spleen	Stomach
Heart	Small Intestine
Kidney	Bladder
Liver	Gall Bladder
Circulation-Sex	Triple-Warmer
Governing	Central

TABLE 1 — **The acupuncture meridians are named according to their associated organs.** Six "hollow" organs, considered yang in quality, are involved in "secretion." Six "solid" organs are described as yin and function in "storage and collection." Thus there are twelve meridian pairs — each meridian pair located symmetrically, one on each side of the body. The final two meridians are single pathways running down the midline of the body: the central meridian (yin) and the governing meridian (yang).

Not only is each organ associated with a bilateral meridian pair, but also with one of the five elements, five seasons, five planets, five colors, and five tastes.

The five-element theory is of central importance to traditional acupuncture theory. All living forms were seen as a mixture of the five elements: Fire, Earth, Metal, Water, and Wood — with each element exhibiting a balance between the yin and yang principles. The expression of these elements in the body is through the flqw of qi along the meridians.

The theory of the five elements, like all Chinese medical philosophy, is process-oriented. In this case, the "mother-son" dynamic is the underlying process:

> The mother-son principle states that as you proceed clockwise, each Element gives birth to the following Element. The ashes of Fire give birth to the Earth. Earth creates minerals, metals, and gems — Metal. Each continues in this way. (Green, 1984, p. 24)

Thus, a blend of the five elements is manifested in the physical world as the five tastes, five colors, and so forth. (See Figure 1.)

The final two meridians in the cycle are single pathways, the central meridian (yin) and the governing meridian (yang), both running through the midline of the body along the spinal cord (Duke, 1972).

When the body is balanced, the vital energy, qi, is flowing freely through the 14 meridians and acupuncture points. The body is in health and harmony; for qi is the regulator of the body's functions, including the blood, nerves, and organs.

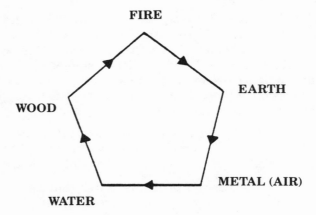

FIGURE 1 — **The five-element theory: the mother-son process.** The five-element theory is process-oriented, each element giving "birth" to the following element. The five elements are manifested in the physical world as the five tastes, five colors, etc.

Disease, then, can be defined in terms of an excess or a depletion of energy along the various yin or yang meridians and associated acupuncture points. In general, an excess of qi is correlated with pain, overheating, and hyperactivity; whereas a depletion of qi is related to cold, numbness, paralysis, and lethargy.

A basic treatment rationale is derived from this excess-depletion principle: tonification-sedation (Mann, 1973). Tonification would be any procedure involved in increasing yang energy, as in a pale, thin patient suffering from chronic fatigue. A sedation technique would be appropriate for a patient with an excess of yang — one who is restless, heavy, reddish in complexion, and has trouble sleeping. The tonification-sedation concept can be applied to a deficiency or excess in yin energy as well.

Various diagnostic techniques are used in traditional acupuncture to determine energy imbalance: inspection of the mouth, nose, eyes, teeth, voice, and breathing. The flow of qi in the meridians is also checked by an examination of radial pulses.

Subtle and complex diagnostic interpretations of the radial arterial pulse were essential to classical Chinese medicine. The *Nei Jing* described over 20 pulses that characterized yin and yang excesses. These pulses were taken at three different depths with three fingers.

In clinical practice, a patient's pulse would actually be made up of a combination of several pulses rather than a single pulse type. However, as an illustration, a pulse having excess yang qualities would be the "rapid" pulse (more than five beats per breath). This pulse pattern would indicate that the "heat" of the body is "accelerating the movement of the 'Blood' " (Kaptchuk, 1983). A pulse pattern showing an excess of yin would be the "slow" pulse (fewer than four beats per breath). This type of pulse would suggest that the "cold" of the body is retarding movement of the "Blood."

After proper evaluation, treatment would then be initiated, usually consisting of a series of acupuncture sessions. Thin, solid needles would be inserted into appropriate yin and yang points to harmonize the qi. When pressure is exerted at these points with the fingers or thumbs, rather than needles, the procedure is termed **acupressure** or **Shiatsu** (in Japan).

Since the meridian network connects not only the organs to various surface loci but also relates the organs to one another, the interrelationships become complex. The key to an effective treatment is in balancing the movement of qi throughout the meridian network, and not merely at the acupuncture points that are manifesting "symptoms."

It is clear from the above descriptions that the ancient Chinese did not base their knowledge on modern human anatomy. In fact, gross dissection of the body was forbidden in a culture that honored its dead. Instead, Chinese medicine is based on an "energetic concept of the body":

> . . . The Chinese system of medicine was based on an energetic concept of the body rather than a material one. In a sense, the early Chinese philosophers anticipated Einstein's theory of relativity, for they recognized that matter and energy were just two different manifestations of the same thing. Rather

than focusing on the material aspects of the body (muscles, nerves, bones, etc.), they concentrated on the vital life energy that creates and animates the physical body. (Bresler, 1981, p. 410)

As foreign as the "energetic" concept of the Chinese may first appear to the contemporary approaches of Western medical science, parallels do exist. For example, yin and yang relationships can be compared to the functional and anatomical branches of the autonomic nervous system: the **sympathetic** and the **parasympathetic.** (See Chapter 17.) Stated simply, overactivity of the sympathetic division, the arousal or "fight or flight" response, has a similarity to the hyperactive functioning characteristic of excessive yang diseases. In turn, overactivity of the parasympathetic portion might be associated with the fatigue in ailments involving excess yin.

Theories of disease and behavioral disorders seen as a function of autonomic imbalances have been proposed by several contemporary Western investigators and will be discussed in Chapter 17.

Although concepts of traditional Chinese medical theory and Western medical science have certain parallels, it would be wrong to draw a one-to-one correspondence. The yin and yang forces should not be considered as a concrete anatomical entity like the construct of the sympathetic/parasympathetic divisions of the autonomic nervous system. As previously mentioned, in the Chinese world view, reality is not seen as discrete, cause-and-effect events. Rather, mental and physical realities are seen as an undulating pattern of primordial energy. This not only makes acupuncture an elegant and profound theory but also a difficult one to translate and evaluate in terms of Western scientific theory and research.

Great emphasis is placed here on traditional Chinese thought and acupuncture theory as an origin of body therapies in general because of the influence and acceptance it has had in the West and throughout the world. Modern acupuncture therapy is used for a variety of medical problems in the Far East, Europe, Britain, the United States, and the Soviet Union.

More than any other form of ancient or contemporary somato-therapy, acupuncture has generated experimental research — especially concerning its use in pain management and anesthesia. (See Chapter 18.)

Many current versions of body therapy have borrowed from or have parallels with ancient acupuncture theory: Reichian therapy (Chapter 10), Polarity (Chapter 11), and Touch for Health (Chapter 11).

REFERENCES

Bresler, D. Chinese medicine and holistic health. In A. Hastings, J. Fadiman, and J. Borden (Eds.), *Health for the Whole Person*. Boulder, CO: Westview Press, 1981.

Chu, L. Yeh, E., and Wood, D. *Acupuncture Manual: a Western Approach*. New York: M. Dekker, 1979.

Duke, M. *Acupuncture*. New York: Pyramid House, 1972.

Green, B. *The Holistic Body Therapy Textbook*. San Diego, CA: Body-Mind Enterprises, 1984.

Kaptchuk, T.J. *The Web That Has No Weaver*. New York: Congdon and Weed, Inc., 1983.

Lao Tzu. *Tao Te Jing* (trans. Chu Ta-Kao). New York: Samuel Weiser, 1972.

Mann, F. *Acupuncture, the Ancient Chinese Art of Healing*. New York: Vintage Books, Random House, Inc., 1973.

Stanway, A. *Alternative Medicine*. New York: Penguin Books, 1979.

Veith, I. *The Yellow Emperor's Classic of Internal Medicine*. Berkeley, CA: University of California Press, 1972.

Watts, A. *The Way of Zen*. New York: Vintage Books, 1957.

Almost every tradition speaks of **kundalini [prana]** in one form or another and describes kundalini in its own way. In Japanese it is called **ki;** in Chinese, **qi;** the scriptures of Christianity call it the **Holy Spirit.**

— Swami Muktananda

CHAPTER 2
THE HATHA YOGA TRADITIONS OF INDIA

The use of postures and breathing exercises for spiritual and physical well-being goes back to the third millennium BC and the Indus valley in India. Here seals were found that portray various physical postures called **asanas** (Worthington, 1982). The first written records of such methods are recorded in sacred Vedic literature, the **Upanishads** (1,500 BC); references are also made in the **Bhagavad Gita** and the Tantric texts, the **Yogacara** and **Vajrayana** (400 BC).

The first detailed description comes from the classic **Yoga Sutras** of Patanjali about 300 BC. Patanjali outlines eight practices or "limbs" of yoga — two of which were the asanas and the pranayama (Wood, 1974). Asanas included any body postures "practiced to strengthen the body, purify the nerves, and develop one-pointedness of mind" (Muktananda, 1978). In the ancient yogic literature, 84 asanas are mentioned. **Pranayama** was defined as a technique of controlling the breath to regulate the flow of prana or "vital energy" through the body (Muktananda, 1979).

As with the Chinese technique of acupuncture, the methods of what later were termed **Hatha yoga** can only be understood in the context of ancient Indian religious thought and metaphysics. Traditionally, Hatha yoga and all yogic practices were methods to assist the individual in achieving a state of enlightenment or self-realization called **samadhi.** The samadhi state, however, was not merely a spiritual state of

13

"mind" but rather a state of psycho-physiological integration, involving a unity of mind and body.

It was not until the tenth century AD that postures and breathing were described separately as a body therapy for preventing disease and maintaining health. During this period, the techniques became associated with classical **Ayurvedic** medicine, a tradition which also has its origin in the Vedic scriptures (Worthington, 1982). Also during this time, the term **Hatha** was first used to describe the physical postures and exercises — "ha" meaning sun and "tha" meaning moon.

Hatha yoga, like acupuncture, is based on the viewpoint of seeing man as an energetic being operating within the larger energy system of the universe. The **prana** or vital energy of the body is considered to be an extension of the same cosmic energy that sustains and directs the universe.

The prana energy flows through a network of channels called **nadis.** There are some 72,000 nadis in the human body that connect it with the universal energy flow; but only three — **ida, pingala,** and **sushumna** — are of importance to yoga (Muktananda, 1979).

The sushumna nadi runs through the core of the body from the sacral region up the spine to the crown of the head. The ida and pingala nadis spiral around the sushumna nadi in an upward direction with the ida terminating in the left nostril and the pingala terminating in the right nostril. The ida is related to the moon and has a "cooling" effect, while the pingala is associated with the sun and has a "heating" effect. This complementary polarity between ida and pingala echoes that of the yin and yang balance found in Chinese thought (Chapter 1).

It is also interesting to note that the traditional symbol of the medical profession, the **caduceus,** appears to be a representation of these three nadis, although its origin is unknown (Worthington, 1982). (See Figure 2.)

Located along the central axis of the sushumna nadi are six energy centers or **chakras** (meaning wheels); a seventh is located above the crown of the head. The chakras, in the yogic traditions, are considered energy centers that transform the universal energy into usable human forms of energy.

Note that the chakras, the nadis, and the flow of universal prana are thought to be in the "subtle" realm and nonphysical in nature, although, as described below, the chakras have physical correlates with the nervous and endocrine systems (Muktananda, 1979; Worthington, 1982). (See Table 2.)

The first chakra, **muladhara,** is located at the base of the spine and is associated with the earth and self-preservation. It is anatomically associated with the sacrococcygeal plexus of the peripheral nervous system and the adrenal glands of the endocrine system.

The second chakra, **svadisthana,** is located just below the navel and is anatomically related to the sacral plexus and the spleen. This chakra is associated with sexual drive and pleasure.

Manipura, the third chakra, is concerned with the individual's sense of ego or personal power. The manipura is correlated with the solar plexus and pancreas and is the regulator of digestion and physical well-being.

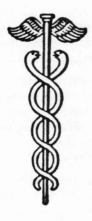

FIGURE 2 — **The caduceus appears to be a representation of the three nadis: the sushumna as the staff and the ida and pingala nadis spiraling around the sushumna as the two oppositely twined serpents.** The caduceus (Latin), meaning the "staff of Mercury," has been the traditional symbol of the medical profession in the West since classical times, although its origin is unknown.

CHAKRA	NERVE PLEXUS	ENDOCRINE GLAND
Muladhara	Sacrococcygeal plexus	Adrenal
Svadisthana	Sacral plexus	Spleen
Manipura	Solar (celiac) plexus	Pancreas
Anahata	Cardiac plexus	Thymus
Vishudda	Laryngeal plexus	Thyroid
Ajna	Cerebellum	Pineal and pituitary
Sahasrara	Cerebral cortex	none

TABLE 2 — **The seven major chakras and their correlates with the nervous and endocrine systems.**

The fourth chakra, the **anahata,** is located in the heart region and is associated with the cardiac plexus and the thymus gland. The anahata is related to the sense of touch, emotions, and the spiritual realm. The energy of the first three lower chakras can be controlled or "sublimated" by the fourth.

Vishudda, the fifth chakra, is situated in front of the throat and is involved in communication and self-expression. It is associated anatomically with the laryngeal plexus and the thyroid gland.

The sixth chakra, the **ajna,** is considered the seat of intelligence, insight, and psychic abilities. It is located between the eyebrows. Anatomically, the sixth chakra is correlated with the cerebellum and the pineal and pituitary glands.

The seventh chakra, the **sahasrara,** is positioned on top of the head and is related to the spiritual world and enlightenment. The sahasrara's anatomical correlate is the cerebral cortex. As the first chakra (muladhara) is the individual's contact with the earth and natural world, the sahasrara is his contact with the spiritual domain.

The purpose, then, of Hatha yoga techniques is to balance the prana flow through the pingala and ida nadis, respectively. Upon the balancing of these two channels, the prana or **Kundalini** energy becomes activated and begins its ascension up the sushumna nadi, piercing the six chakras to the seventh, the sahasrara.

> When awakened, Kundalini begins to move upward within the sushumna, the subtle central channel, piercing the chakras and in-

itiating various yogic processes which bring
about total purification and rejuvenation of
the entire being. When Kundalini enters the
sahasrara, the spiritual crown of the head,
the individual self emerges in the universal
Self and attains the state of Self-realization
or Samadhi. (Muktananda, 1978, p. 301)

As previously stated, the balancing of the prana flow
through the nadis and chakras occurs in the "subtle,"
nonphysical realm, but corresponding events are manifested in the physiology of the physical or "gross" body.
The 72,000 nadis are associated with the blood vessels,
nerves, and lymph ducts; while the chakras, as mentioned, are correlated with nerve plexi and endocrine
glands. Thus, as the prana through the channels is balanced, the body's physiology is also brought into harmony or "homeostasis" (Kuvalayananda and Vinekar,
1979).

In fact, much of Hatha yoga was eventually integrated
with Ayurvedic medicine. Ayurvedic practice is one of
the oldest known healing systems, having its origins,
like yoga, in the Vedic scriptures (Thakkur, 1974).

According to Ayurvedic practice, each patient can be
classified as being predominated by mucus, fire, or
wind — or different combinations of the three. This
classification is considered the person's "constitution."

The mucus humor, or **kapha,** is the "structural" humor
associated with **anabolic** activity in the body such as
tissue growth and repair. In Western medical science,
it may be anatomically correlated with **parasympathetic** activity of the autonomic nervous system.
(See Chapter 17.)

The fire or **pitta** humor, is associated with heat or **catabolic** processes such as the breaking down of sugars. Pitta is most likely correlated with **sympathetic** autonomic function.

The **vata,** or wind humor, represents the "nerve currents" of the body, including the endocrine glands. The wind humor appears anatomically correlated with the spinal cord and brain (i.e., the **central nervous system**).

The central purpose of Ayurvedic medicine is to balance the three humoral or energetic qualities. Hatha yoga became integrated with other modes (herbal medicines and diet) to achieve such harmony.

For example, a patient that had a depletion of fire humor might have the "peacock" asana prescribed to stimulate catabolic (e.g., digestive) secretions. Another patient having an excess of fire disposition might be given the "lotus" position to stimulate anabolic secretions. Along with these yoga postures, appropriate diet and herbal remedies would also be prescribed (Das and Satsang, 1978).

In Hatha yoga, we see again a somatic technique that is intricately woven into the religious and metaphysical thought of the culture. And later, Hatha yoga became assimilated and integrated into Ayurvedic medicine. Both had their origins in the sacred scriptures of India, the Vedas, and are sometimes referred to as "sister sciences."

Like Chinese acupuncture — Hatha yoga, with its energetic concepts of prana, chakras, and humoral balances — has reappeared in modern forms of body therapy: Rolfing (Chapter 9), Polarity (Chapter 11) and Therapeutic Touch (Chapter 11).

REFERENCES

Das, B.H., and Satsang, D.S. Ayurveda: the yoga of health. In E. Bauman, A.I. Brint, L. Piper, and P.A. Wright (Eds.), *The Holistic Handbook*. Berkeley, CA: And/Or Press, 1978.

Kuvalayananda, S., and Vinekar, S.L. Principles of yogic therapy. In D.S. Sobel (Ed.), *Ways of Health*. New York and London: Harcourt Brace Jovanovich, 1979.

Muktananda, S. *The Play of Consciousness*. San Francisco: Harper and Row, 1978.

Muktananda, S. *Kundalini: the Secret of Life*. Ganeshpuri, India: Gurudev Sidda Peeth, 1979.

Thakkur, C. *Introduction to Ayurveda*. New York: ASI Publishers Inc., 1974.

Wood, E.E. *Practical Yoga, Ancient and Modern*. Hollywood, CA: Wilshire Book Co., 1974.

Worthington, V. *A History of Yoga*. London: Routledge and Kegan Paul, 1982.

Disease [is] not an entity, but a fluctuating condition of the patient's body, a battle between the substance of disease and the natural self-healing tendency of the body.

— *Hippocrates*

CHAPTER 3
CLASSICAL GREEK, ROMAN, AND OTHER EARLIER INFLUENCES

Early Origins from Other Cultures

Although detailed descriptions are beyond the scope of this book, it should be mentioned that somato-procedures appeared in many ancient cultures. Manipulation and massage practice were found in early Hebrew, Egyptian, Mesopotamian, Persian, and Japanese medical practices.

As an illustration, an ancient Egyptian papyrus, written about 1,700 BC, portrayed an impressive knowledge of the relation between spinal alignment and proper muscular functioning:

> If thou examinest [a man having] a sprain in a vertebra of the spinal column, thou shouldst say to him "Extend now thy legs [and] contract them both [again]." When he extends them both he contracts them both immediately because of the pain he causes in the vertebra of his spinal column in which he suffers. (Breasted, 1930)

After making this diagnosis, adjustment of the displaced vertebra by means of massage and manipulative procedures (both spinal and soft tissue) was then made by the Egyptian physician.

The use of touch as a mode of healing was recorded in the writings of the Hebrew and Christian traditions. The "laying on of hands" was particularly prominent

25

in first-century Christianity. Full body massage with oils goes back even further in Jewish practices (Krieger, 1979; Kelsey, 1973).

The ancient Mayan people of Central America and the Incas of South America also utilized methods of joint manipulation and massage (Venzmer, 1972).

Therefore, touch as a method of healing cannot be traced or attributed solely to one or two ancient cultures but appears to have developed from multiple origins, global in scope.

Classical Greek and Roman Influences

Somato-methods, including massage and musculo-skeletal manipulation, were evident in Greek culture as early as 1,500 BC. One early Greek papyrus described the movement and manipulation of legs and pelvis in the treatment of lower back pain. Whether these techniques spread from the Far East or developed regionally is not known.

By the fifth century BC, the Greek physician Herodicus was recommending the use of exercise and massage for medical purposes (Tappan, 1980).

Hippocrates (460–357 BC), a student of Herodicus and later known as the "Father" of scientific medicine, gave significant attention to the techniques of massage and spinal manipulation (Venzmer, 1972).

Of the 70 books attributed to Hippocrates, two dealt specifically with the use of somato-therapies in medical practice: *Manipulation and Importance to Good Health* and *On Setting Joints by Leverage.*

Hippocrates suggested the use of massage strokes for various muscle-skeletal problems, including the following procedures for a dislocated shoulder:

> It is necessary to rub the shoulder following the reduction of a dislocated shoulder. It is necessary to rub the shoulder gently and smoothly. (Soloman, 1950, p. 521)

The Hippocratic writings also showed an awareness of the consequences that different degrees of massage pressure have on muscle and the surrounding tissues:

> Hard rubbing binds, much rubbing causes parts to waste and moderate rubbing causes them to grow. (Peterson, 1946)

Furthermore, Hippocrates also saw a relationship between the spine and the onset of disease:

> Get knowledge of the spine, for this is the requisite of [understanding] many diseases. (Peterson, 1946)

For Hippocrates, harmony with nature resulted in health, while discord led to disease. His writings stressed the natural recuperative power of the body itself—encouraging proper diet, rest, exercise, and hygiene as well as massage and manipulation to enhance the natural healing process. Very few drugs were recommended, for according to Hippocratic medicine:

> . . . to prescribe nothing is sometimes an excellent medicine. (Venzmer, 1972, p. 78)

In 46 BC, a Greek physician of the Hippocratic tradition, Asclepiades, was granted Roman citizenship and became the first of many outstanding Greek physicians to teach and practice in Rome. Asclepiades found the traditional Hippocratic system of medicine too passive in its approach and developed an alternative consisting largely of body therapies. His treatments included massage techniques which he believed restored the "nutritive fluids" of the body to their natural free movement (Tappan, 1980). Asclepiades was the first Western physician to note the relationships between types of touch or **tactile stimulation** and their physiological consequences. For instance, he is credited with the discovery that light stroking applied to the back region will induce sleep. (See Chapter 17.)

Another Roman physician of Greek origin, Claudius Galen (130–200 AD), generally considered the greatest anatomist and physiologist of classical times, was also known to employ spinal adjustments to the vertebrae. Galen, for example, once corrected a paralysis of the right arm by adjusting the cervical vertebrae (Wilk, 1973).

The somato-practices of the classical Greeks and Romans were in part the forerunners of several contemporary musculoskeletal techniques. Their use of massage, joint manipulation, and spinal adjustments can now be found in modern chiropractic (Chapter 7) and osteopathic (Chapter 6) methods and theories.

REFERENCES

Breasted, J.H. (trans.). *The Edwin Smith Surgical Papyrus* (Vol. 1). Chicago: University of Chicago Press, 1930.

Kelsey, M. *Healing and Christianity.* New York: Harper and Row, 1973.

Krieger, D. *The Therapeutic Touch.* Englewood Cliffs, NJ: Prentice Hall, Inc., 1979.

Peterson, W.F. *Hippocratic Wisdom: For Him Who Wishes to Pursue Properly the Science of Medicine.* Springfield, IL: Charles C. Thomas, 1946.

Soloman, W.M. What is happening to massage. *Archives of Physical Medicine,* 1950, 521–523.

Tappan, F.M. *Healing Massage Techniques.* Reston, VA: Reston Publishing Co., 1980.

Venzmer, G. *Five Thousand Years of Medicine.* (Trans. by Marion Koenig.) New York: Taplinger, 1972.

Wilk, C.A. *Chiropractic Speaks Out.* Park Ridge, IL: Wilk Publishing Co., 1973.

I was astounded, and often no less mortified, at the number and variety of instances in which the bonesetters' [treatments] I have endeavoured to describe were followed by almost immediate cure.

— *Wharton Hood*

CHAPTER 4
FROM THE DARK AGES TO MODERN TIMES

With the decline of the Roman Empire, healing through touch diminished in Western medicine. This was due, in part, to the destruction of numerous libraries by invaders as well as to repressive actions taken by the orthodox Christian Church during the "Dark Ages."

The Church saw manipulative procedures as being of "demonic" origin. During the Middle Ages, many healers were burned at the stake for demonic possession and witchcraft. Mark Twain in his short novel, *The Mysterious Stranger*, portrays the following scene from 16th century Austria:

> It was bitter cold weather when Gottfried's grandmother was burned. It was charged that she had cured bad headaches by kneading the person's head and neck with her fingers—as she said—but really by the Devil's help, as everybody knew. (Twain, 1962, p. 340)

Yet certain somato-techniques (e.g., spinal manipulation and the laying on of hands) persisted throughout most of Europe. The procedures were performed mostly by unschooled physicians, lay healers, and priests.

It was not until the 16th century that the brilliant French surgeon, Ambroise Pare, began to employ massage techniques again for joint stiffness and wound healing after surgery (Venzmer, 1972). Pare delineated three types of massage strokes: gentle, medium and vigorous. Pare is credited with creating the anatomical and physiological foundations for physical medicine in the West.

It was also during the Renaissance that spinal and soft-tissue manipulation regained public popularity for various musculoskeletal problems. The practitioners were known as "bonesetters" and by the 17th century had gained a wide following in Europe (Grossinger, 1980). The art and science of bone setting was handed down from father to son like other trades and skills of the time. Unlike their Greek and Roman predecessors, the bonesetters were typically from the uneducated classes: barbers, blacksmiths, and the like.

The medical establishment of Europe and later the United States largely ignored their work. For with the advent of the biomedical period in Western science and medicine, body therapy remained in the background until the latter half of the 19th century.

REFERENCES

Grossinger, R. *Planet Medicine*. Garden City, NY: Anchor/Double-day, 1980.

Twain, M. *The Mysterious Stranger*. Boston: Houghton Mifflin Co., 1962.

Venzmer, G. *Five Thousand Years of Medicine*. (Trans. by Marion Koenig.) New York: Taplinger, 1972.

Is it not reasonable to suppose that, if one form of skin stimulation [massage] can produce muscular contraction by reflex, another form can secure relaxation.

— *James B. Mennell*

CHAPTER 5
SWEDISH MASSAGE: PER HENRIK LING

The experimental discoveries concerning biology and medicine by Harvey in the 17th century and Muller, Bernard, and Pasteur in 18th and 19th centuries ushered in the biomedical period. Somato-therapies were still in the background.

It was, however, the emerging science of physiology in the early 19th century that allowed Per Henrik Ling to put forth a theory of massage techniques that to the present is widely accepted (Lawrence and Harrison, 1983).

Ling was a Swedish instructor of fencing and gymnastics. His interest in massage started with "rheumatism" in his arm and shoulders. He developed a system of massage that utilized many of the positions and movements of Swedish gymnastics. With a combination of these massage strokes and exercises, he successfully remedied his ailment. His system was based on the newly discovered knowledge of the circulation of the blood and lymph. (See Chapter 13.) Ling's concepts became known as the "Ling System" or "Swedish Movement Treatment" (Tappan, 1980).

There are five primary strokes in **Swedish massage** procedures (see Figure 3):

1. **Effleurage,** or "stroking," involves long, centripetal strokes to the legs, arms, back, and trunk. It is used to increase the general circulation as well as blood flow to the area being worked.

35

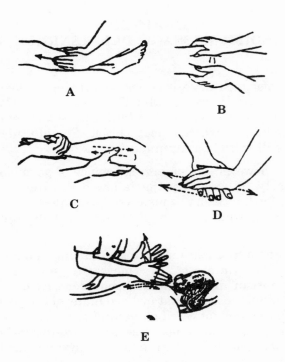

FIGURE 3 — **Five basic Swedish massage strokes:** (A) effleurage to the leg; (B) petrissage to the knee; (C) friction stroke to the forearm; (D) vibration stroke to the back; and (E) tapotement to the back.

2. **Petrissage,** or "kneading," includes the wringing, squeezing, and rolling of muscles to stimulate lymphatic flow and deep blood flow and to relax hypertoned muscles.
3. **Tapotement,** or "percussion," is used to enhance muscular and neural function by cupping or tapping with the hands.
4. **Vibration** involves a shaking movement to the tissues with the hand and is also thought to stimulate the nervous system.
5. **Friction** massage is accomplished by deep circular movements to the joints and around boney prominences. It is used for the breaking down of scar tissue and adhesions.

Initially, Ling's system was rejected by the Swedish government and the medical community. In 1813, with the support of influential clients, he was granted a license to practice and teach his method, establishing the Royal Gymnastic Central Institute. By the time of Ling's death in 1839, Swedish massage had obtained worldwide recognition.

Institutes of massage appeared in France, Germany, and Austria by the mid-19th century. People suffering from various musculoskeletal problems sought out these spas. The treatments consisted of massage, mineral baths, and exercise (Tappan, 1980).

By the early 20th century, Swedish massage techniques had been revised and accepted in both England and the United States. In 1911, massage was first used in modern times by an English orthopedic surgeon, Sir Robert Jones, for the treatment of fractures.

James B. Mennell, another Englishman and a contemporary of Jones, summarized the effects of massage in two categories: **mechanical** and **reflex** actions (Mennell, 1917).

Under mechanical action, Mennell refers to four ways that massage exerts a mechanical effect:

1. Assisting in venous return of blood to the heart
2. Aiding lymph movement out of the tissues
3. Stretching of the connective tissue (e.g., tendons, scar tissue, etc.)
4. Mechanical stimulation of the stomach, small intestine, and colon

Concerning the reflex action of massage, Mennell maintained that certain forms of tactile stimulation (e.g., stroking, light touch, etc.) stimulated reflex arcs, causing muscles to relax or contract according to the type of stroke applied. (See Chapter 16.) He proposed, ahead of his time, that both smooth and skeletal muscles were under the control of such reflexes:

> . . . we know from nature and our own experience that this stroking massage is capable of yielding comfort, and yet is so light that its effects cannot be conceivably due to mechanical causes: the only possible way, therefore, in which it can act is by nerve reflex. Moreover, we all recognize certain reflexes that result from skin stimulation—the abdominal, plantar, and cremasteric reflexes. We also recognize the involuntary emptying of the stomach on touching the back of the throat. . . . Is it not reasonable to suppose that, if one form of skin stimulation can pro-

duce muscular contraction by reflex, another form of stimulation can secure relaxation. (Mennell, 1917, p. 5).

Mennell also cited clinical examples involving orthopedic surgery and the reduction of pain that resulted from massage following such surgery.

The mechanical and reflex effects of massage that Ling, Mennell, and others observed are now supported by experimental research and will be discussed in detail in Part II of this book.

In 1913 an American physician, William H. Fitzgerald, introduced a massage method called **Zone therapy** or **Reflexology** (Ingham, 1959). Similar to the energetic concepts of Chinese acupuncture, reflexology speaks of "zones" along the body that affect the flow of energy to the various organs. The zones end in the feet, where points can be stimulated to produce a "reflex" action in a corresponding zone (i.e., organ or other anatomical structure). (See Figure 4.)

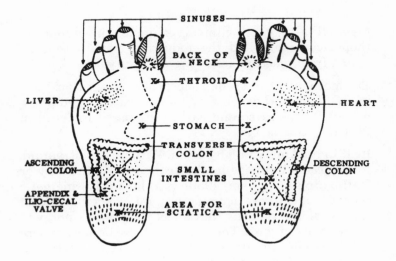

FIGURE 4 — **Reflexology or Zone therapy.** Reflex points for the major organs, glands and other structures on the soles of the feet. The exact mechanism and pathway for these "reflexes" are still in question.

REFERENCES

Ingham, E.D. *Stories the Feet Can Tell: Stepping to Better Health.* Rochester, NY: E.D. Ingham, 1959.

Lawrence, D.B. and Harrison, L. *Massageworks.* New York: Putnam Publishing Group, 1983.

Mennell, J.B. *Massage: Its Principles and Practice.* London: Blakiston's Son and Co., 1917.

Tappan, F.M. *Healing Massage Techniques.* Reston, VA: Reston Publishing Co., 1980.

... the fascia is the place to look for the cause of disease and the place to consult and begin the action of remedies of all diseases.

— *Andrew Taylor Still*

CHAPTER 6
OSTEOPATHY: ANDREW TAYLOR STILL

Andrew Taylor Still (1828–1917) was a practicing country doctor in the state of Missouri when he founded and developed the theory and manipulative techniques of osteopathy.

Still had lost three of his children to spinal meningitis. It was this tragedy and the common misuse of powerful toxic drugs of the era that led to his rejection of orthodox medicine.

Influenced by his engineering background, Still proposed that structural problems in the body are behind most disease processes. If the structural relationships within the body become distorted, a corresponding physiological dysfunction will occur: "structure determines function." Any structural abnormality that causes an illness was termed an "osteopathic lesion" (Still, 1899). The term is misleading in that the Greek **osteo** means "bone" and **pathos,** "disease;" and osteopathic lesion was not intended to refer only to "bone diseases."

Still studied the anatomy of animals and primates in terms of evolutionary directions. He pointed out that vertebrates, like man and other primates, have just recently begun to walk on two feet. This change from a quadruped to a biped has put considerable stress on the intravertebral discs by making them bear weight. Similarly, the development, according to Still, of a vertical stance displaced the organs downward causing

43

hernias, constipation, back problems, etc. (Solit, 1962). (See Figure 5.)

The key to eliminating osteopathic lesions and thus returning the body to balance and health was circulation. In 1870, Still defined the "rule of the artery":

> Whenever the circulation of the blood is normal, disease cannot develop because our blood is capable of manufacturing all the necessary substances to maintain natural immunity against disease. (Still, 1899)

The rule of the artery implied more than mere blood flow through the major arteries. Still believed in a "fluid continuity" throughout the body (Frymann, 1980). This circulatory balance involved:

1. The movement of blood from the heart to the periphery (body extremities)
2. The lymphatic drainage from the peripheral tissues back into the venous system to the heart
3. The adequate movement of the cerebrospinal fluid in the brain and spinal cord

Thus, proper physiological and structural function of the body was seen as dependent on the fluid continuity among the various tissues and organs.

As traditional Chinese acupuncture theory considered the flow of qi or vital energy necessary for harmonious functioning, Still believed that proper fluid circulation was essential. (See Chapter 1.)

Also as in Oriental medicine, Still thought health had several diminsions of expression. He referred to the "total lesion" as involving three levels of body function-

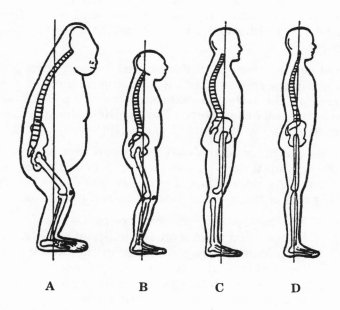

FIGURE 5 — **The development of the erect posture in primates:** (A) gorilla, (B) Neanderthal man, (C) "average" man, (D) "balanced man." Note the overall curvature of the spine goes from a "C" shape in the gorilla to an "S" curve in the "balanced" man.

ing: biochemical, structural, and psychological. Remedying the total lesion involved working at all three levels simultaneously; this was called a "total adjustment."

Osteopathic lesions were removed by bony manipulations of the spine and soft tissues around the joints. An area on the body that exhibited the signs of a lesion was typically characterized by swelling, thickened connective tissue, and pain (Deason, 1913).

Still and his students also recognized that balance in the nervous function, as well as proper circulation, was crucial. As osteopathic theory developed, the controlling role of the nervous system gained importance:

> The osteopathic lesion . . . rests for its interpretation upon a broad biological basis. It is fundamentally a blockage of the afferent [sensory] impulse. And any interference with the afferent integrity means disorder, disease, for thereby growth, development, repair of tissue and vital resistance is impaired. The body being built upon mechanical lines is subject to maladjustment whether bone, muscle, ligament or viscus, and this at once implies interference with the afferent impulse and as a result the . . . whole is deranged. (Deason, 1913, p. 377)

For Still, the connective tissues, particularly the fascial sheaths, were the underlying structural component behind the dynamic unity among the body's systems:

> . . . fascia is . . . a foundation on which to stand. By its action we live and by its failure

we shrink or swell or die. The soul of man
with all the streams of pure, living water
seems to dwell in the fascia of his body. (Still,
1899, p. 162)

He felt that the integrity of the fascial wrappings
around the body's organs, muscles, and nerves was essential in understanding and remedying disease:

... the fascia is the place to look for the
cause of disease and the place to consult and
begin the action of remedies of all diseases.
(Truhlar, 1950, p. 54)

An early student of Still's William G. Sutherland, developed the concept of "cranial" osteopathy about the
turn of the century. Sutherland observed a rhythmic
contractive and expansive articular motion in the cranial bones (Sutherland, 1939). He called this oscillation
the "primary respiratory mechanism" that resulted
from the cerebro-spinal fluid's fluctuating pressure on
the dural membranes of the spinal cord. In a sense, it
can be thought of as a basic rhythm of the central nervous system:

This primary respiratory mechanism includes the brain, the intracranial membranes, the cerebro-spinal fluid and the articular mobility of the cranial bones; and also
the spinal cord, the interspinal membranes,
again the cerebro-spinal fluid and the articular mobility of the sacrum between the ilia.
(Sutherland, 1939, p. 2)

Normally, the primary respiratory rhythm is palpated
between 8-12 cycles per minute. Sutherland and others

have defined health and disease in terms of variations in the amplitude, the symmetry, and the frequency of the "cranio-sacral" pulse (Upledger and Vredevoogd, 1983). Recently some osteopathic investigators have correlated the cranio-sacral rhythm with the Traube-Herring wave, a slow wave of 6-15 cycles per minute associated with the electrical activity of the heart (Frymann, 1980).

Contemporary osteopathy appears more like orthodox, allopathic medicine than the manipulative therapy of Still and his students. Modern osteopaths use pharmacological agents extensively as well as surgery. In the United States, many states use the same licensing requirements for osteopaths (D.O.'s) and M.D.'s. Manipulation and many of Still's concepts, however, are taught in the osteopathic medical schools. In addition, other body therapists (e.g., Rolfing practitioners) have adopted and developed some osteopathic procedures.

REFERENCES

Deason, J. *Physiology: General and Osteopathic.* Kirksville, MO: The Journal Printing Co., 1913.

Frymann, V.M. The expanding osteopathic concept. *Journal of Energy Medicine,* 1980, *1,* 86–91.

Solit, M. Study in structural dynamics. *Journal of the American Osteopathic Association,* 1962, *62,* 30–40.

Still, A.T. *Philosophy of Osteopathy.* Published by A.T. Still, 1899.

Sutherland, W.G. *The Cranial Bowl.* Mankato, MN: W.G. Sutherland, 1939.

Truhlar, R.E. *Doctor A.T. Still in the Living.* Privately published, 1950.

Upledger, J.E., and Vredevoogd, J.D. *Craniosacral Therapy.* Chicago: Eastland Press, 1983.

There is an inborn, innate intelligence in every living being, and in every plant that grows. Innate [intelligence] uses the nervous system through which to transmit its orders. . . .

— Daniel David Palmer

CHAPTER 7
CHIROPRACTIC: DANIEL DAVID PALMER

The word chiropractic comes from the Greek words **cheir,** "hands," and **praktikos,** "done by"—that is, "done by hands."

The chiropractic technique of spinal manipulation was created by Daniel David Palmer in 1895. Palmer was a self-educated beekeeper, fish peddler, and grocer from Iowa. Prior to developing the chiropractic method, he was involved in lay healing for nine years using "animal magnetism." Throughout this period, he studied numerous books on anatomy and physiology, with his focus concerning the human spine and spinal nerve transmission (Bach, 1968).

Palmer performed his first successful spinal adjustment on a janitor who had a hearing problem. The janitor told Palmer that he had experienced 17 years earlier a "give" in his back and since then had had a hearing defect. Palmer then palpated the upper thoracic spine and made a vertebral adjustment. After this "specific adjustment," the man could "hear as before":

> Harvey Lillard, a janitor in the Ryan Block, where I had my office, had been so deaf for 17 years that he could not hear the racket of a wagon on the street or the ticking of a watch. I made inquiry as to the cause of his deafness and was informed that when he was exerting himself in a cramped, stooped position, he felt something give way in his back

51

and immediately became deaf. An examination showed a vertebra racked from its normal position. I reasoned that if that vertebra was replaced, the man's hearing should be restored. . . . I racked it into position by using the spinous process as a lever and soon the man could hear as before. (Palmer, 1910)

Palmer believed, like the Oriental philosophers, in an "innate intelligence" within all living matter which governed its existence. He considered the nervous system to be, physiologically, the "control system" over the body's as well as the mind's functions:

There is an inborn, innate intelligence in every living being, and in every plant that grows. Innate uses the nervous system through which to transmit its orders. . . . Innate has all to do with control of the vital functions, and through them, indirectly, the control of the intellectual functions. (Altman, 1981, p. 57)

While Still's (osteopathic) emphasis was on the "rule of the artery" and the proper circulation of the bodily fluids, Palmer thought disease resulted when the normal transmission of nerve impulses was impeded.

Impulses are made in the brain and connected with the body by a system of nerves through which this force passes in currents. . . . Functions are names given to these actions, any interference to the passage of these vitalizing currents produces abnormal functions—disease. (Altman, 1981, p. 48)

This inhibition of the neural impulses was thought to be caused by an impingement upon the nerve root at the point where it passes out of the intervertebral foramen. The intervertebral foramen is created by the articulations of the vertebrae above and below it. Such a condition Palmer defined as "subluxation":

> ... a condition in which one of the vertebra has lost its juxtaposition with the one above or below to an extent less than a luxation [a severe misalignment of the joint] that occludes an opening, impinges on nerves and interferes with normal neurological function. (Stephenson, 1948, p. 16)

Thus, Palmer saw the proper exiting of the nerve roots from the intervertebral foramen as essential to the control of bodily functions: digestion, glandular, circulation, locomotion, respiration, etc. (See Figure 6.)

The purpose, then, of the spinal adjustment was to correct the subluxation, restoring normal neural activity which in turn would allow a return to proper functioning of the various organs and physiological mechanisms.

Palmer, it should be noted, recognized that spinal adjustments had a long history before his discovery:

> I am not the first person to replace vertebrae, but I do claim to be the first to replace displaced vertebrae by using transverse and spinous processes as levers.... (Palmer, 1910, p. 29)

Palmer's manipulative approach emphasized a quick thrust of the specific vertebrae, which is in contrast to

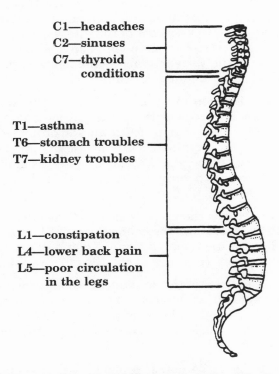

C1—headaches
C2—sinuses
C7—thyroid
    conditions

T1—asthma
T6—stomach troubles
T7—kidney troubles

L1—constipation
L4—lower back pain
L5—poor circulation
    in the legs

FIGURE 6 — **Spinal adjustments and physiological function.** In chiropractic theory, subluxation of a vertebra causes impingement and compression on spinal nerve roots. Some of the problems associated with given vertebral misalignments are outlined above.

the osteopathic method of Still. Still's work was a more generalized technique involving pressure, traction, and stretching of the soft tissues that attach to the bony skeleton. (See Chapter 6.)

As the popularity of Palmer's work spread, the Palmer Infirmary and Chiropractic School was established in Davenport, Iowa, in 1897.

In 1907, his son, Bartlett J. Palmer, took over and largely directed the course of chiropractic work as a profession. For most of his life, B.J. Palmer was involved in controversy with the medical establishment as well as his fellow chiropractors. He believed that chiropractic spinal adjustments should be performed solely with the hands, although diagnosis could include non-touching procedures. B.J. Palmer introduced the first use of X-rays in the detection of spinal analysis.

Following the death of D.D. Palmer in 1913, chiropractic grew rapidly although it had continual opposition from the American Medical Association (AMA). Since 1974, however, chiropractic care has been recognized by Medicare, Worker's Compensation programs, and many insurance companies as valid health care.

Contemporary chiropractic theory is divided into two schools. The orthodox ("straights") school keeps to Palmer's notion that the vertebral subluxation is the fundamental cause of disease, and treatment should be restricted to adjustment of the spine. The unorthodox ("mixers") school has expanded the scope of chiropractic to include any treatment (physical therapy, nutrition, vitamins, etc.) that enhances the "natural" healing mechanisms of the body.

A popular technique used by the unorthodox group involves muscle testing, called "applied kinesiology" or "Touch for Health" (Goodheart, 1982; Thie, 1979). This method synthesizes chiropractic theory with the energy-meridian theory of classical Chinese acupuncture. Muscles are identified with a given meridian and organ. (See Chapter 1.)

Whether a given muscle tests weak or strong indicates the condition of that meridian and organ. Treatment involves the "tonification" or strengthening of a weaker muscle which, in turn, allows a relaxing or "sedation" of a stronger muscle. Yet more than "muscles" are being treated:

> Using applied kinesiology, the muscle balancing technique, we will be testing for specific muscle weakness and treating them. You should realize, however, that we are not just treating muscles. The body is one thing, a coherent whole, with many different systems and functions. (Thie, 1979, p. 11)

Therefore, in chiropractic techniques and theory, the traditions of spinal manipulation from the classical Greeks and the Chinese system of energy channels are both clearly in evidence.

REFERENCES

Altman, N. *The Chiropractic Alternative*. Los Angeles: F.P. Tarcher, Inc., 1981.

Bach, Marcus. *The Chiropractic Story*. Los Angeles: DeVorss, 1968.

Goodheart, G.J. Reactive muscle patterns in athletes. *ACA Journal of Chiropractic*, 1982, *16*, 45–59.

Palmer, D.D. *The Science, Art, and Philosophy of Chiropractic*. Portland, OR: Portland Printing House, 1910.

Stephenson, R.W. *Chiropractic Textbook*. Davenport, IA: Palmer School of Chiropractic, 1948.

Thie, J.F. *Touch for Health*. Marina del Rey, CA: DeVorss, 1979.

When I was experimenting with various ways of using myself . . . , I discovered that a certain use of the head in relation to the neck and of the neck in relation to the torso . . . constituted a **Primary Control** of the mechanisms as a whole.

— *F. Mattias Alexander*

CHAPTER 8
ALEXANDER TECHNIQUE:
F. MATTIAS ALEXANDER

In the 1890's, a young Australian actor and monologist, F. Mattias Alexander (1869–1955), developed a technique of body re-education designed to improve the use and alignment of the body (Alexander, 1969; Barlow, 1980).

For Alexander, the method evolved out of treating a personal difficulty: the recurring loss of his voice while performing. After observing his problem with the aid of a three-way mirror, he noticed that the voice loss was related to a backward and downward movement of his head. By inhibiting this pattern of pressure on the back of the neck, Alexander found that his voice limitations disappeared. Furthermore, he experienced an overall positive effect on his body's functioning. He wrote the following account:

> After I had worked on this plan for a considerable time, I became free from my tendency to revert to my wrong habitual use in reciting, and the marked effect of this on my functioning convinced me that I was at last on the right track, for once free of this tendency, I also became free from throat and vocal trouble and from respiratory and nasal difficulties which I had experienced from birth. (Jones, 1976, p. 18)

From the success of experience, Alexander developed a broad philosophy and method concerning learning and human activity. The actual technique was based on the principle of inhibiting habitual, inefficient movements, thereby allowing new creative choices of motor activity to occur.

In 1904 he took his method to England, and some years later to the United States with the help of his younger brother, A.R. Alexander. Between 1910 and 1941 F.M. Alexander published four books describing the philosophy and procedures of his work. Since his death in 1955, his teachings and techniques have been spread by instructors and training schools throughout the world.

The technique itself involves an upward lengthening of the spine with special attention focused on the head and neck alignment, a relationship which Alexander termed "primary control." (See Figure 7.)

Frank Pierce Jones, a student of Alexander who later conducted experimental studies concerning the technique, defined primary control as:

> ... the dynamic relation of the head and neck that promotes maximal lengthening of the body and facilitates movement throughout the body. Physiologically it is the stimulus (head-neck relation) which serves to activate the antigravity reflexes. (Jones, 1976, p. 166) (See also Chapter 16.)

Through both subtle manipulative touch and verbal feedback, the "student" is encouraged to inhibit habitual movements or stereotyped responses, permitting the free choice of more efficient movement. This

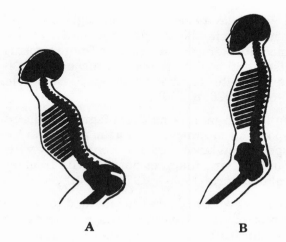

A   B

FIGURE 7 — **Primary control: the dynamic relation of the head and neck that "promotes maximal lengthening of the body."** In (A) the subject lacks this relationship as he moves towards a sitting position, while in (B) the same subject is exhibiting the lengthening process.

delaying of habitual motor response Alexander called "inhibition."

> If you delay response long enough to inhibit neck muscle shortening, it prevents an immediate stereotyped response from imposing itself and facilitates making a choice that is appropriate to the situation as a whole. (Jones, 1976, p. 150)

> Inhibition maintains the integrity of the responding organism so that a particular response can be carried out economically without involving inappropriate activity from unrelated parts. (Jones, 1976, p. 149)

Alexander never considered his method to be a form of therapy or medical treatment. Rather, he saw it as a way of educating the person, allowing him to choose new options of thinking as well as of movement. Again, in the words of Jones:

> Alexander was frequently accused by the medical profession of claiming to cure disease. He always denied the charge. What he claimed was that the use of the technique raises the general health level and that the results in some cases had astonished him. These included cases of paralysis, tuberculosis, asthma, "incipient appendicitis," and colitis. . . . The "cures" were significant because they illustrated the general principle. Alexander promised his pupils that if they learned the technique, all motor habits would be broken up and "an improved efficiency would follow as a matter of

course." . . . In other words the technique is not curative but preventative. (Jones, 1976, p. 35)

Alexander's philosophy echoes that of the ancient Greek physician Hippocrates, who believed that the body and mind as a totality must be taken into account rather than symptoms or disease processes alone:

The nature of the body must be regarded as a whole in every consideration of the medical art. (Peterson, 1946, p. 202)

REFERENCES

Alexander, F.M. *The Resurrection of the Body.* New York: Delta, 1969.

Barlow. W. *The Alexander Technique.* New York: Warner Books, Inc., 1980.

Jones, F.P. *Body Awareness in Action.* New York: Schocken Books, Inc., 1976.

Peterson, W.F. *Hippocratic Wisdom: For Him Who Wishes to Pursue Properly the Science of Medicine.* Springfield, IL: Charles C Thomas, 1946.

. . . many therapies are striking at the pattern of disease, instead of supporting the pattern of health.

When the body gets working appropriately, the force of gravity can flow through. Then spontaneously, the body heals itself.

— Ida P. Rolf

CHAPTER 9
ROLFING: IDA P. ROLF

Ida P. Rolf (1896–1979) was born in New York City. In 1920 she received her Ph.D. in biological chemistry from Barnard College and then worked at the Rockefeller Institute (now Rockefeller University) for the next several years (Connelly, 1977).

In 1928 her father died, and she resigned from the Rockefeller Institute to settle family affairs. It was during this period that Rolf gave up her research interests in chemistry and began the development of her manipulative method, **Structural Integration,** or later to be known as **Rolfing.**

By the late 1930's she was quite familiar with osteopathy, chiropractic, Alexander technique, Hatha yoga, and homeopathic medicine. Like many of her predecessors, part of Rolf's interest in body and touch-oriented therapies came from her own health problems and later her family's:

> I had plenty wrong with me; I was a curvature case, but I didn't know it. And I was a prediabetic [hypoglycemic] and I didn't know that either. (Feitis, 1978, p. 6)

Although she sought out practitioners with various methods, she felt that their techniques were inadequate to deal with her difficulties.

Rolf studied and was significantly influenced by Andrew Still's osteopathic theory—particularly with the premise that structure creates and determines

67

physiological function. (See Chapter 6.) She was impressed with osteopathy's use of soft-tissue manipulation (i.e., fascia and tendons) around joints for the relief of stress and injury. Yet she considered this kind of "local work" merely shifting the physical strain to another area of the body:

> When you force a locally misaligned area into line, you only shift the strain. The strain above and below that local area is still the same; it has shifted a little bit. There is no basic change in function. You go on using that body in the same way you always used it, and the strain goes right back to the same place. (Feitis, 1978, p. 171)

Rolf was convinced that the entire structural order of the body needed to be realigned and balanced with the gravitational forces in order for permanent "changes" to occur. She used the term "random bodies" to refer to the result of physical and emotional traumas: a fall down the stairs, a bicycle accident or overbearing parents.

While Palmer's chiropractic, and to a lesser extent Still's osteopathy, emphasized the manipulation of bony processes of the spine, Rolf directed her intervention towards the myofascial system (i.e., the muscles, tendons, ligaments, and surrounding connective tissue). In Rolf's theory, these soft tissues represent the structural organ of the body and are highly "plastic" in quality:

> The idea of the chiropractors and before them some of the osteopaths is that the basic problem of the body is in the bony struc-

ture . . . We say that the bony spine is a secondary index; the spine is where it is by vir-
tue of where we align the myofascial structure which is the connective tissue system.
Fascial connective tissue is the organ of
structure. Fascial layers comprise the layers
of structure, the organ that holds the body in
the three dimensional world. . . . This organ
of structure is a very resilient, elastic, plastic
medium. It can be changed by adding energy.
(Feitis, 1978, p. 177)

Rolf's contributions to the field of somato-therapy include not only her use of connective-tissue manipulation, but also her recognition of gravity's effect on body
structure and function:

Stress, aches, and pains are the body's language to express the strain and imbalance
between the field of gravity and the body's
integrals—weight masses of the head,
thorax, pelvis, and legs. Such a body is unbal-
anced; we call it random. Return to balance
is possible. Manipulation to reposition the
soft tissues will give a greater freedom to
muscles. This can be combined with a pat-
terning of freer movement to achieve more
appropriate balance. (Rolf, 1973, p. 7)

Although Rolf firmly believed that the myofascial tissues were the medium to induce structural change in
the body, she also stressed the effects the method had
on the nervous system, especially the role of the autonomic nervous system:

It is interesting to note that some osteopathic
researchers believed that the health of the
joints reflects the well or ill of the autonomic
nervous system rather than the newer central nervous system. The difference between
these two systems will manifest in behavior
and offers one clue to change in behavior patterns elicited by Rolfing. (Rolf, 1976, p. 13)

The functioning of the musculoskeletal system was considered inseparable from the outflow of the autonomic
nervous system.

In addition to osteopathy and chiropractic, Rolf studied
the "asanas" (i.e., postural positions) of Hatha yoga.
Like the yogic philosopher-healers of ancient India, she
believed that somato-therapy would not only enhance
physical structure but also emotional and spiritual
"well-being." In fact, much of her early work included
yoga positions with their emphasis on increasing joint
space by stretching (Feitis, 1978). (See Chapter 2.)

Following the energetic model of "chakras" found in
yogic traditions, Rolf described the myofascial network
as a pathway through which "energy seems to flow":

If you accept the idea of energy centers, the
idea if you want to call them that, of chakras,
you know that the one absolutely reliable
way of enhancing that energy is not by dealing with the chakra per se, . . . but by dealing
with the myofascial system, the system along
which energy seems to flow through. . . .
(Rolf, 1976, p. 16)

By the late 1950's, Rolf had developed her soft-tissue manipulative technique into a sequence of ten-hour sessions, each session having specific goals. (See Figure 8.) For example, the first session involved opening the chest, shoulders, and hip joint; while the second session included work on the feet, legs, and back. The sequence continued through the body's myofascial tissue, working from the outer superficial layers to the deeper layers. The final three sessions were concerned with integrating the earlier work. Additional sessions and "advanced series" were also available.

Until the late 1960's, Rolfing was virtually unknown except by chiropractors, osteopaths, and other therapists that Rolf had taught. At this time, Rolfing was "discovered" by psychologist Fritz Perls at the Esalen Institute in Big Sur, California. In 1970 the Rolf Institute of Structural Integration was established in Boulder, Colorado, to supervise training and research. Rolfing practitioners are now found in Europe as well as the United States.

The reported therapeutic effects of Rolfing cover a wide spectrum of medical and psychological benefits. Yet like F.M. Alexander (Alexander technique), Rolf maintained that Rolfing was a method of "education" and "supporting the pattern of health," rather than a therapy that deals with disease per se:

> So many therapies are striking at the pattern of disease, instead of supporting the pattern of health. One of the things that you as Rolfers must always emphasize is that you are not practitioners curing disease; you are practitioners invoking health. (Feitis, 1978, p. 202)

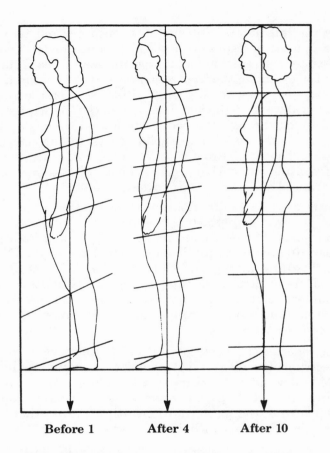

Before 1   **After 4**   **After 10**

FIGURE 8 — **The Rolfing method.** The above three illustrations were traced from photographs of a client undergoing the ten sessions of the Rolfing technique: before the first session, after the fourth, and after the tenth. Note how the segments of the head, thorax, pelvis, and legs are progressively restored to a vertical alignment with the gravitational field.

REFERENCES

Connelly, L. Ida Rolf. *Human Behavior,* 1977 (May), 17–23.

Feitis, R. *Ida Rolf Talks about Rolfing and Physical Reality.* New York: Harper and Row, Publishers, 1978.

Rolf, I.P. A contribution to the understanding of stress. *Confinia Psychiatrica,* 1973, *16,* 69–79.

Rolf, I.P. Dr. Ida P. Rolf's 1976 Annual Meeting Message. *Bulletin of Structural Integration,* 1976, *5,* (Dec.), 8–16.

. . . we must trust not only the character attitudes but also the muscular attitudes corresponding to them. This causes part of the work to be shifted from the psychological . . . to the immediate dissolution of the muscular armor.

— *Wilhelm Reich*

CHAPTER 10
REICHIAN THERAPY: WILHELM REICH

Wilhelm Reich, an Austrian psychoanalyst, was a clinical assistant to Sigmund Freud for six years. He became interested in the physiological basis of neurosis. By the late 1920's, his radical and controversial theories concerning sexuality led to his separation from Freud. In 1934, Reich settled in the United States.

Reich is considered by many to be the founder of psychotherapeutic body techniques (Hoff, 1978). While classical psychoanalytic theory was verbal and insight-oriented, Reich's body therapy of "character analysis vegetotherapy" focused directly on the physiological realms which he assumed were underlying psychological character.

Reich defined "character structure" as a person's "habitual attitudes and consistent patterns of response to various situations" (Reich, 1973). Each type of psychological defense of the "ego" was associated with a specific biological pattern of muscular tension. For example, sadness might be disguised behind a constant, pleasant smile on the level of character structure and by restricted musculature on a less-visible somatic level. These "constellations" of muscular tension Reich termed "muscular armor."

Gradually he moved the emphasis of his therapeutic approach away from the psychological to the realm of the physical body:

> . . . we must trust not only the character attitudes but also the muscular attitudes cor-

responding to them. This causes part of the work to be shifted from the psychological and character realms to the immediate dissolution of the muscular armor. (Reich, 1973, p. 299)

Reich developed many somato-techniques to dissolve the muscular armor. His therapy had seven major stages which were intended to release the body's somatic defenses from the most superficial to the deepest:

1. Deep breathing with the intent of producing emotional and autonomic release
2. Deep muscular massage to areas of chronic spasticity while the client breathes deeply
3. Working with facial expressions and sounds—combining them with deep breathing
4. Pushing down on the chest as the client exhales to release the breathing muscles
5. Stimulating the gag reflex or cough reflex for deep internal armoring
6. Maintaining "stress positions" while breathing or expressing with the voice or face
7. Asking the client to produce various movements: kicking, stamping, etc.

The goal of Reichian therapy was to dissolve neurotic psychological structure and muscular armoring at their deepest physiological levels. Specifically, this involved for Reich the liberation of the "libidinal" or sexual energy to establish "full orgastic potency":

> There can be no doubt, therefore, that the highest and most important goal of . . . therapy is the establishment of orgastic potency, the ability to discharge accumulated

sexual energy completely. (Reich, 1973, p. 112)

He believed that full orgastic potency concerned a person's ability to build up the body's "charge" and subsequently to release or "discharge" this energy through sexual orgasm:

> . . . Orgastic potency is to surrender to the flow of biological energy, to free inhibitions: the capacity to discharge completely the stored up sexual excitation through involuntary, pleasurable convulsions of the body. (Reich, 1973, p. 102)

As Reich began to insist that all neuroses and even physical disease were caused by the inability of the individual to enjoy unblocked sexual orgasm, his work was largely rejected by his psychoanalytic peers.

Expanding his theory, Reich decided that the inability to express sexual energy (i.e., "sexual stasis") had its effect on the "vegetative" or autonomic nervous system:

> "Sexual stasis" means nothing other than an inhibition of vegetative [autonomic] expansion and blocking of the activity and motility of the . . . vegetative organs. (Reich, 1973, p. 348)

According to Reich, sexual stasis was a root cause in any disease process.

Reich viewed the sexual energy of the body as having a dynamic pulsating character. The balanced individual should oscillate between two poles: "expansion" and "contraction." He associated the parasympathetic branch of the autonomic nervous system—the nurturing activities of digestion, sexuality, etc.—with the expansive pole. Likewise, the sympathetic division—the activities of arousal and "fight or flight," etc.—were correlated with the contractive aspect (see Chapter 17):

> . . . all biological impulses . . . can be reduced to **expansion** (elongation, dilation) and **contraction** (shrinking, constriction) . . . How are these two basic functions related to the autonomic nervous system? Investigation of the complicated vegetative innervations of the organs show that the parasympathetic (vagus) always functions where there is expansion, dilation, hyperemia, turgor and pleasure. Conversely, the sympathetic nerves function whenever the organism contracts, blood is withdrawn from the periphery, and pallor, anxiety, and pain appear. (Reich, 1973, p. 288)

When the body's energy is blocked or inhibited, muscular armor will build up concurrently with a pattern of neurotic character structure. He called such a person "chronically contracted," which physiologically involved a constant sympathetic response—"sympatheticotonia" (Reich, 1973).

As found in Eastern philosophy, Reich saw a unity between mind and body, psychological and physical aspects:

> Mind and body constitute a functional unity, having at the same time antithetical relationships. (Reich, 1973, p. 379)

Like the Taoist view of ancient China, man and the universe were seen as an oscillating pattern of contraction ("yang") and expansion ("yin"). The Chinese called this vital energy that is behind the pattern "qi"; Reich called it "orgone energy." (See Chapter 1.)

While the Chinese considered the vital energy as nonphysical in nature, Reich was convinced that the orgone energy was detectable and measurable. Reich's later work involved experiments to measure and accumulate orgone energy for healing purposes (Reich, 1951).

However, Reich came increasingly into conflict with the medical establishment. He was eventually investigated by the U.S. Food and Drug Administration and was prosecuted and convicted for fraudulent medical practices. In 1957, Reich died while serving his sentence in federal prison.

Reich's earlier ideas and therapy have greatly influenced contemporary body work. A popular somatotherapy that evolved directly from his system is **Bioenergetics.** Bioenergetics was founded by Alexander Lowen, an American psychiatrist and a student of Reich's for twelve years (Lowen, 1975).

REFERENCES

Hoff, R. Overview of Reichian therapy. In E. Bauman, A.I. Brint, L. Piper, and P.A. Wright (Eds.) *The Holistic Handbook.* Berkeley, CA: And/Or Press, 1978.

Lowen, A. *Bioenergetics.* New York: Penguin Books, Ltd., 1975.

Reich, W. *The Orgone Accumulator—Its Medical and Scientific Use.* London: CORPS, 1951.

Reich, W. *The Function of Orgasm.* New York: Farrar, Straus, and Giroux, 1973.

We act in accordance with our self-image. This self-image—which, in turn, governs our every act—is conditioned in varying degree by three factors: heritage, education, and self-education.

— *Moshe Feldenkrais*

CHAPTER 11
OTHER CONTEMPORARY BODY THERAPIES

Many other contemporary somato-systems that involve touch have appeared in this century. Several of the more influential methods will be briefly discussed below.

Polarity Therapy

In the early 1900's, Polarity therapy was created by an American physician, Randolph Stone (Gordon, 1983). Stone studied numerous body systems, both ancient and modern: acupuncture, Hatha yoga, osteopathy, chiropractic, and reflexology. From his investigations, he concluded that a "magnetic field" regulated and directed the physiological systems of the body. Influenced by Oriental philosophy and medicine, Stone believed all aspects of the universe to be expressed in opposite poles (e.g., male-female, positive and negative electrical charges, etc.); hence, he called his therapeutic method "Polarity." (See Chapter 1.)

The Polarity therapist utilizes four basic approaches in restoring balance to the magnetic patterns around and within the body:

1. Development of a positive mental attitude
2. Application of gentle pressure to points on the skin, releasing the body's blocked energy flow
3. Instruction in Polarity yoga or movement to further balance and vitalize the body

4. Education in a proper diet consisting of fresh fruits, vegetables, and other whole foods

The Feldenkrais Method

In the 1940's, the mathematician and physicist Moshe Feldenkrais was influenced by F.M. Alexander's concept of body re-education: the inhibiting of habitual movement and allowing free choice of more efficient patterns (Feldenkrais, 1970, 1972). (See Chapter 8.)

Feldenkrais' method utilizes touch, postural adjustments, and exercises to reintegrate the neuromuscular system. The key is the development of a greater awareness of "body image" and associated movements. This new awareness is accomplished by breaking down movements into smaller components, which is thought to in turn establish new neural connections between the motor cortex of the brain and the muscular system—connections that have become "short circuited" through bad habits and physical trauma.

Laying on of Hands

Laying on of hands (i.e., placing the hands on the body with the intention to heal) is a form of therapy that is found in Judeo-Christian traditions as well as in other ancient cultures. Throughout the history of Christianity, silent and spoken prayer has been combined with touch as a healing technique. (See Chapter 4.)

Presently, this tradition is widely in use in the Christian "renewal" movement. The following passage describes the healing of a 19-year-old woman in Colombia, South America, through the laying on of hands or "soaking prayer":

> Shortly after her visit to the doctor, a group gathered again . . . for further prayer. As we laid hands on Teresa we noticed that the place where the bone was broken was quite warm and the lump greatly reduced in size. We prayed for about two hours and finally . . . asked Teresa to stretch her leg and foot. . . . She felt no pain or discomfort as she moved her leg. We were all thankful and joyful, for it seemed as if the bone had welded. However, we advised Teresa to see a doctor before she used her leg. Several days later she saw not one but two doctors, both of whom confirmed that her bone had welded. (MacNutt, 1977)

Dolores Krieger, nurse and researcher, has demonstrated in controlled studies that the use of intentional and empathetic   touch can raise blood hemoglobin values in hospital patients (Krieger, 1975). (See Chapter 13.) She refers to her laying on of hands technique as **Therapeutic Touch.**

Basic Movement

The fields of modern dance and basic movement have also produced methods of somato-therapy (Aston, 1980; Wing, 1982; Sweigard, 1974). As might be expected, the focus is on how the human body moves and interacts within its environment; but guiding touch and manipulation are also employed.

The techniques for movement created by Rudolf Laban and expanded on by Irmgard Bartenieff serve as an excellent illustration (Bartenieff, 1980). Following Reich's idea of "muscular armor," Bartenieff assumes that a person's psychological and physiological states are represented and reflected in his postural-movement patterns. A combination of movement, breathing, and manipulative touch is utilized to break down these patterns, permitting the individual new choices in how he carries and moves himself.

REFERENCES

Aston, J. A somatics interview with Judith Aston. *Somatics,* 1980 (Autumn), 8–11.

Bartenieff, I. *Body Movement: Coping with the Environment.* New York: Borden and Breach, 1980.

Feldenkrais, M. *Body and Mature Behavior: A Study of Anxiety, Sex, Gravitation and Learning.* New York: International Universities Press, 1970.

Feldenkrais, M. *Awareness Through Movement.* New York: Harper and Row, 1972.

Gordon, R. *Your Healing Hands: The Polarity Experience.* Berkeley, CA: Wingbow Press, 1983.

Krieger, D. Therapeutic Touch: the imprimatur of nursing. *American Journal of Nursing,* 1975, *75,* 784–787.

MacNutt, F. *The Power to Heal.* Notre Dame, Indiana: Ave Maria Press, 1977.

Sweigard, L.E. *Human Movement Potential.* New York: Dodd, Mead, and Co., 1974.

Wing, H. Rolfing movement integration: movement education for everyday life. *Bulletin of Structural Integration,* 1982, *8* (Spring-Summer), 1–9.

Rather than focusing on the material [structural] aspects of the body, they [Oriental physicians] concentrated on the vital life energy that creates and animates the physical body.

— *David E. Bresler*

CHAPTER 12
NOTHING NEW UNDER THE SUN

The history of healing through touch is a story that tends to repeat itself.

From the Far East evolved somato-systems based on an **energetic** concept—the balancing of "qi" or "prana." This universal, vital energy moves through the body and determines the quality of physiological and psycho-spiritual function. Energetic body therapies include acupuncture and acupressure from China and Japan, and Hatha yoga from India.

From the Western world developed somato-techniques with a **structural** orientation—viewing structural integrity of the spine, the head/neck, and the soft tissues as the key to balanced function. The Greek system of massage/manipulation, Swedish massage, osteopathy, chiropractic, Alexander technique, and Rolfing all emphasize anatomical-structural aspects of body work.

Some contemporary therapies have combined the energetic and structural approaches. Reichian therapy, Polarity, and Therapeutic Touch are examples.

Nearly all modern body systems—whether energetic, structural or a combination—have richly borrowed from ancient traditions of the East and West. In the words of the biblical adage from Ecclesiastes:

> What has happened will happen again, and what has been done will be done again, and there is nothing new under the sun. Is there anything of which one can say, 'Look, this is

new'? No, it has already existed, long ago before our time. The men of old are not remembered, and those who follow will not be remembered by those who follow them. (Ecclesiastes 1:9–11)

PART II
PHYSIOLOGICAL EVIDENCE

Whenever the circulation of the blood is normal, disease cannot develop because our blood is capable of manufacturing all the necessary substances to maintain natural immunity against disease.

— *Andrew Taylor Still*

CHAPTER 13
CIRCULATION OF BODILY FLUIDS

Overview

Circulation, meaning "to pass around," involves the transport of fluids through the body's tissues and organs. The functions of circulation include:

1. Transporting oxygen and nutrients into the tissues
2. Removing carbon dioxide and other waste products from the tissues
3. Protecting the body from infection
4. Assisting in the regulation of body temperature

The two primary fluids involved in these functions are **blood** and **lymph.**

Blood moves through a network of arteries, veins, and capillaries that permeates the body's tissues. The **arteries** carry blood away from the heart. The smallest branches of the arteries terminate in **capillaries.** It is through the capillaries that oxygen and other nutrients are delivered to the tissues and waste products and carbon dioxide are removed. The capillaries end in **veins** that return the blood to the heart. (See Figure 9.)

The fluid that becomes lymph is derived essentially from **blood plasma** that has filtered out of the blood capillaries into the spaces between the cells. The lymphatic circulation originates in capillary-like vessels, although slightly larger. These lymph capillaries are dead-end vessels and form an intricate network within the connective tissue that surrounds the various organs. The lymphatic capillaries converge to form larger

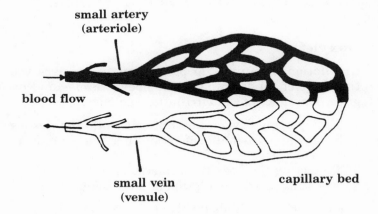

small artery
(arteriole)

blood flow

small vein
(venule)

capillary bed

FIGURE 9 — **The capillary network.** It is through the capillaries that oxygen and nutrients are delivered to the tissues and carbon dioxide and waste products are removed. Somato-procedures appear to produce an opening, or **vasodilation,** of these capillary vessels (see next section).

lymphatic vessels. The waste materials (bacteria, particles, etc.) in the lymph are filtered through plexuses of lymphatic tissue called **lymph nodes.** Lymph nodes are located in the neck, chest, armpits, abdomen, and groin regions. The larger lymph vessels return the lymph into the venous system. The movement of lymph is partly dependent on the contractions of the skeletal and smooth muscles. Backward flow is prevented in the lymph vessels (and also in the veins) by one-way valves.

From ancient times, somato-practitioners have recognized the central importance of touch in promoting balance in the bodily fluids.

Beginning with Harvey's landmark work on the circulatory system, the proper flow of blood and lymph became basic to manipulative massage therapy. By the earlier 1900's, the work by Ling, Jones, and Mennell concerning therapeutic massage was known in the medical community. (See Chapter 5.) Much of the experimental work that examined the effects of **tactile** (touch) procedures on the arterial, venous, and lymphatic circulation was conducted during the first third of this century.

Tactile Procedures and Arterial Blood

Light massage was found to produce a transient opening, or **vasodilation,** of capillary vessels, thereby increasing the peripheral blood flow. Deeper massage strokes produced longer periods of vasodilation (Carrier, 1922). (See also Chapter 17.)

Massage strokes have also been associated with an increase in the total quantity of blood flow through the area under stimulation and a corresponding **systemic** (i.e., total) increase in red blood cells and hemoglobin production (Scott, 1917).

More recently, Krieger (1975) found that the simple act of "laying on of hands" (Therapeutic Touch) by nurses on or close to the body (but not necessarily near the injury or disorder) increased the hemoglobin levels in hospital patients. (See Chapter 11.) The control and experimental groups were comparable for sex, age group, and pre-test hemoglobin levels. The experimental group was treated by nurses "who included treatment by therapeutic touch while caring for their patients; the control group . . . included nurses who gave nursing care to their patients without using the therapeutic touch."

Post-test showed a statistically significant increase in hemoglobin values for the experimental group receiving the laying on of hands. There was no significant difference between pre- and post-test values for the control group.

Touch and Venous and Lymphatic Movement

The mechanical consequences of tactile pressure and squeezing the soft tissues were reported to enhance the venous return of blood to the heart (Landis, 1933). This effect can clinically be observed by deep stroking the superficial veins in the direction of the venous flow (i.e., towards the heart).

Clinical observation also indicates that deep pressure and massage are useful in enhancing lymphatic flow:

> Massage can encourage lymphatic flow, preventing edema that often occurs with inactivity. Since lymph is viscid and moves slowly, massage strokes should be slow and rhythmical. . . . Massage is an excellent mechanical substitute when normal muscular functioning has been interrupted . . . (Tappan, 1980, p. 19)

In one animal study, massage to a dog's foreleg was shown to increase the rate of lymph flow. However, active exercise was found to be more efficient than the passive somato-stimulation for increasing lymphatic movement (Ladd, Kottke, and Blanchard, 1952).

Therapeutic Benefits

The above-cited studies provide strong evidence for the therapeutic usefulness of touch in enhancing circulatory function. The effects may be summarized as follows:

1. Local increases in the dilation of arterial and venous capillaries
2. Systemic increases in blood hemoglobin levels and thus a rise in the supply of oxygen to the tissues and organs
3. Assists in returning the blood through the veins and back to the heart
4. Assists the flow of lymph back into the venous system, reducing excess fluids (i.e., **edema**) in the peripheral tissues

A final benefit of somato-procedures concerns the reduction of chronic pain and inflammation in joints and muscles. Cailliet (1977) proposed that various conditions and traumas (e.g., physical, emotional, infection, immobilization) irritate surrounding muscular tissue, causing an increase in "muscle tension" (contraction). This heightened tension in turn reduces the local circulation to and from this area, inducing **ischemia,** that is, a reduction in blood flow (Travell, 1983).

The ischemia can lead to edema, retention of waste products, and eventually inflammation. If the inflammation becomes chronic, limited joint movement due to the thickening of the fascial connective tissue can result. (See Chapter 14.) It appears that the use of somato-interventions will stop this sequence of events by increasing the regional arterial blood flow as well as by aiding in the removal of wastes via the lymphatic and venous circulation. (See Figure 10.)

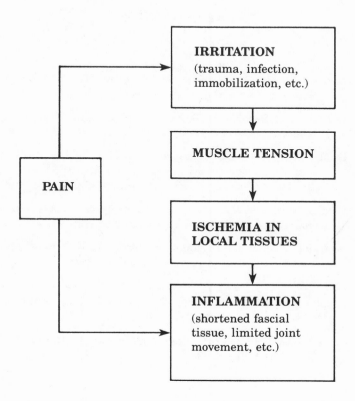

FIGURE 10 — **Joint and muscle pain caused by ischemia (reduced circulation).** Note that somato-interventions break up this sequence of events by increasing the local arterial blood flow.

REFERENCES

Cailliet, R. *Soft Tissue Pain and Disability.* Philadelphia: F.A. Davis Co., 1977.

Carrier, E.B. Studies on the physiology of capillaries. *American Journal of Physiology,* 1922, *61,* 528.

Krieger, D. Therapeutic Touch: the imprimatur of nursing. *American Journal of Nursing,* 1975, *75,* 784–787.

Ladd, M.P., Kottke, E.J., and Blanchard, R.S. Studies of the effect of massage on the flow of lymph from the foreleg of the dog. *Archives of Physical Medicine,* 1952, *33,* 604–612.

Landis, E.M. and Gibbon, J.H. Physiology of venous return. *Journal of Clinical Investigations,* 1933, *12,* 105.

Scott, F.H. Factors influencing the interchange of fluid between blood and tissue spaces. *American Journal of Physiology,* 1917, *44,* 298.

Tappan, F.M. *Healing Massage Techniques.* Reston, VA: Reston Publishing Co., 1980.

Travell, J.G. *Myofascial Pain and Dysfunction.* Baltimore: Williams and Wilkins, 1983.

One wonders the extent to which the cooperative, integrative, communicative, transductive properties of the [connective tissue's] ground substance may serve to order and integrate the rapid and subtle activities of the living system.

— *James L. Oschman*

CHAPTER 14
THE CONNECTIVE TISSUE NETWORK

Overview

Of the tissues found in the human body, connective tissue is by far the most abundant; yet it is the least studied in modern medical science. The connective tissue forms the "organ" of structure and support for the body's other components, creating a continuous network throughout the body.

Connective tissue consists of cells called **fibroblasts,** that are surrounded in a semifluid gel called the **ground substance** or **matrix.** Within this ground substance are (1) fibrous elements composed mainly of **collagen** and **elastic** fibers, and (2) an interfibrillar substance, or cement, consisting largely of complexes of glycoproteins and associated polysaccharides.

The amount of water contained within the connective tissue is apparently related to the condition of the ground substance. For instance, stress, trauma, and aging are associated with decreases in the total water volume within the matrix (Oschman, 1981).

Recent research concerning the body's microstructure indicates that this extracellular ground substance is linked through proteins to the cytoplasm within the cells (Oschman, 1984).

There are six primary types of connective tissue: fascia, tendons, ligaments, cartilage, muscle, and bone, all of which originate from fibroblast cells. Important to this discussion is **fascia.** Fascia is the collagen fibrous web that forms sheaths which surround and penetrate the muscles, organs, blood vessels, and nerves (Junqueria, Carneiro, and Contopoulos, 1977). (See Figure 11.)

Connective tissue serves a variety of functions:

1. Supports the body's tissues and organs and maintains the body's shape and structure
2. Facilitates movement between adjacent structures (e.g., tendon across a bone)
3. Assists the circulation through the veins and lymphatic vessels
4. Participates in tissue repair
5. Retains fluids involved in tissue nutrition

Connective Tissue's Ability to Change Shape

Manipulation and stretching of the fascial sheaths and tendons have long been used as a method of breaking down scar tissue and increasing range of motion in the joints.

How deep tactile pressure produces these often remarkable results is now beginning to be understood. The key is connective tissue's underlying quality of **plasticity**—its capacity to change shape when deep pressure is administered.

Rolf (1977), a biochemist and founder of the soft-tissue manipulative method called Rolfing (Structural Integration), proposed that the properties of fascial connective tissue can be altered by the application of mechanical pressure. (See Chapter 9.) Rolf proposed that a transition occurred in the ground substance of fascia:

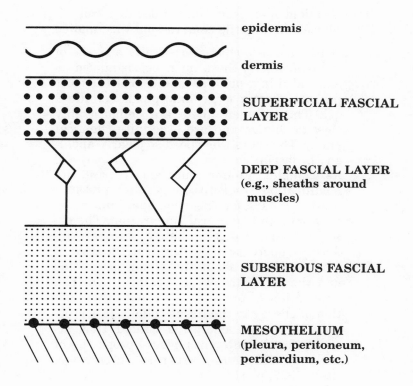

epidermis

dermis

SUPERFICIAL FASCIAL LAYER

DEEP FASCIAL LAYER (e.g., sheaths around muscles)

SUBSEROUS FASCIAL LAYER

MESOTHELIUM (pleura, peritoneum, pericardium, etc.)

FIGURE 11 — **Layers of fascia.** Fascial connective tissue forms a collagen fibrous network throughout the body. Its sheaths surround and penetrate the muscles, organs, blood vessels, and nerves.

from a colloid "gel" (semisolid state) to a "sol" (liquid-like) phase when tactile compression was applied:

> While fascia is characteristically a tissue of collagen fibers, these must be visualized as embedded in ground substance. For the most part, the latter is an amorphous semifluid gel. The collagen fibers are demonstrably slow to change and are a definite chemical entity. Therefore, the speed so clearly apparent in fascial change must be a property of its complex ground substance ... and its modification under changes of pressure would account for the wide spectrum of effects seen in Structural Integration. The observable speed of the changes that are induced supports this hypothesis in the light of what we know about the action of colloids and the physical laws governing them. The application of pressure is, in fact, the addition of energy to the tissue colloid. It is probably this more energized colloid that accounts for the different physical properties of the body undergoing Structural Integration. (Rolf, 1977, p. 41)

There is considerable support for Rolf's position. Many organic gels (e.g., ground substance) "do undergo solation with great readiness" when pressure is applied (Oschman, 1981). After the pressure is released, the organic substance will return to a semisolid state (i.e., "re-gel") at a rapid speed.

A striking illustration of this phenomenon comes from marine biological research concerning the ground substances of the amoeba and the sea urchin. When hydrostatic pressure was experimentally increased, the viscosity (thickness) of the ground matrix decreased, thereby changing the physical shape of these organisms (Brown and Marsland, 1936). In addition to pressure, other forces such as electrical fields have been reported to induce this gel-to-sol transition.

On the molecular level, it appears to be the glycoprotein structure of the ground matrix that breaks down with the addition of heat produced by mechanical compression. This in turn allows the ground substance to change to the sol or liquid-like state (Oschman, 1981). When the pressure is released, the matrix "reshapes" and returns to a "transformed" gel or semi-solid phase. This transformation also involves an increase in the water molecules associated with the proteins in the ground substance (i.e., **hydration**):

> If tissue responds to stress, disuse, or lack of movement by a dehydration of the ground substance (an idea that is supported both by scientific evidence and by the experiences of many body workers), the application of pressure could bring about a rapid solation and rehydration. Removal of the pressure would allow the system to re-gel, but in the process the tissue would be transformed both in its water content and its ability to conduct energy and movement. (Oschman, 1981, p. 25)

Connective Tissue as a Conductor of Electrical Charge

It has been demonstrated that the connective-tissue network is capable of conducting weak electrical currents in response to pressure or stretching of tendons, muscles, and ligaments (Fukada, 1974). This property of a crystalline material (e.g., connective-tissue proteins) producing electrical fields when compressed is termed the **piezoelectric effect** (Becker and Selden, 1985).

It has been further hypothesized that the semi-conductor properties of protein macro-molecules found in connective tissue might involve the movement of electrons along the proteins themselves. Furthermore, the movement of charged particles (i.e., current) would be dependent on the amount of water associated with the proteins (Gascoyne, Pethig, and Szent-Gyorgyi, 1981).

Perhaps in addition to the integrated circuits of the nervous system, there exists a second communication network in the body through the web of connective tissue carrying a flow of electrons.

Such a concept certainly might help explain the actual physical pathway or channels of energy movement described in many of the somato-therapies: the "meridians" of acupuncture and the "chakras" and "nadis" of Hatha yoga. The exact nature and anatomical location of these channels has long been in question. (See Chapters 1 and 2.)

Therapeutic Benefits

Certainly clinical and experimental evidence indicate that connective tissue can be altered through deep tactile pressure and stretching. This has several practical applications:

1. Treating muscular "contractures" following long periods of immobility (e.g., bone fractures)
2. Increasing the range of motion in joints after muscle strain or joint sprain
3. Breaking down of scar tissue caused by trauma (e.g., whiplash or surgery)

Soft-tissue manipulative therapy appears to be particularly useful in treating these connective-tissue-related problems.

In a study involving ten cerebral palsy patients, classified as having "mild," "moderate" or "severe" impairment, a series of Rolfing manipulative sessions was adminstered (Perry, Jones, and Thomas, 1981). The subjects were evaluated before and after the treatments for velocity, stride length, cadence during walking, and for general muscle strength and muscular electrical activity. It was found that velocity, stride length, and cadence improved in the mild group and velocity in the moderate group. No significant changes were reported in the severe group. The investigators concluded that the Rolfing method may be an appropriate treatment for cerebral palsy patients that "have the neurological capacity to use the increased mobility."

The writer encountered similar findings in a clinical study of six individuals having mild cerebral palsy. All six underwent a sequence of Rolfing sessions. Pictures and clinical assessments were made before and after the treatments. Four of the six individuals showed marked improvement in walking patterns and standing posture (Cottingham, 1981). (See Figure 12.)

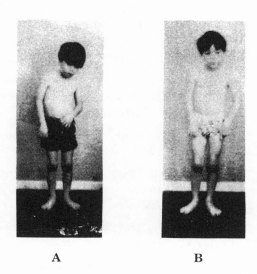

A   B

FIGURE 12 — **Rolfing technique as a treatment for cerebral palsy.** Profile view of a five-year-old boy with mild, spastic cerebral palsy. Photographs were taken before the first session (A) and after the fifth session (B) of the Rolfing method. As well as the postural changes, the boy's gait pattern (walking) noticeably improved.

REFERENCES

Becker, R.O., and Selden, G. *The Body Electric.* New York: Morrow, 1985.

Brown S., and Marsland, D.A. The viscosity of amoeba at high hydrostatic pressure. *J. Cell Comp. Physiol.,* 1936, *8,* 159–165.

Cottingham, J.T. Unpublished study concerning the effects of Rolfing on mild, spastic cerebral palsy, 1981.

Fukada, E. Piezoelectric properties of organic polymers. *Ann. N.Y. Acad. Sci.,* 1974, *238,* 7–25.

Gascoyne, P., Pethig, R., and Szent-Gyorgyi, A. Water structure-dependent charge transport in proteins. *Proc. National Academy of Science,* 1981, *78,* 261–265.

Junqueria, L.C., Carneiro, J., and Contopoulos, A. *Basic Histology.* Los Altos, CA: Lange Medical Publications, 1977.

Oschman, J.L. *The Connective Tissue and Myofascial Systems.* Berkeley, CA: Aspen Research Institute, 1981.

Oschman, J.L. Structure and Properties of Ground Substances. *American Zoologist,* 1984, *24,* 199–215.

Perry, J., Jones, M.H., and Thomas, L. Functional evaluation of Rolfing in cerebral palsy. *Develop. Med. Child. Neural.,* 1981, *23,* 717–729.

Rolf, I.P. *Rolfing: The Integration of Human Structures.* Santa Monica, CA: Dennis-Landman Publishers, 1977.

The brain and spinal cord of mammals, including man, consist of some billions of neurons, and a single neuron may connect with thousands of others. How is this enormous . . . network organized?

— *Walle H. Nauta*

CHAPTER 15
THE NERVOUS SYSTEM

Overview

The nervous system is the regulator or controller of bodily processes, modulating the functions of the organs and tissues.

Functionally, the nervous system has three primary responsibilities:

1. It receives and filters information from the internal and external environment.
2. It integrates this information (i.e., "defines" the stimulus).
3. It then responds to this stimulus with some form of output.

The fundamental unit of the nervous system is the single nerve cell, the **neuron.** The neuron is composed of: (1) a cell **body,** (2) **dendrites** that receive impulses from other neurons or sense organs, and (3) an **axon** that sends nerve impulses to dendrites of other neurons. (See Figure 13.)

The intersection between two neurons, where the impulse is transferred, is called a **synapse.**

The actual nerve impulse, or **action potential,** is coded in the movement of ionic charge along the membrane of the neuron. It thus is an electrochemical event.

The nervous system is made up of a network or "integrated circuit" of neuron units. The simplest nervous system is found in certain polyps and sea anemones,

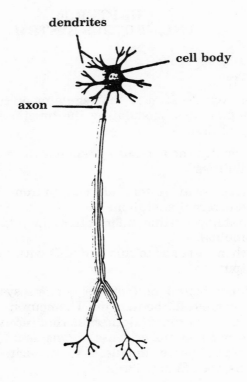

FIGURE 13 — **The neuron is the fundamental unit of the nervous system:** the dendrites which receive nerve impulses; the cell body of the neuron; and the axon which in turn sends impulses to other neurons.

consisting of a single neuron (Nauta and Feirtag, 1979). The dendrite of this neuron transmits sensory data to its cell body, while its branching axon sends motor information into a contractile fiber. This neural pathway by which a sensory stimulus in some part of the body is translated into movement is called a **reflex arc.**

The next level of organization of the reflex arc is the two-neuron system found in certain polyps and jellyfish: a **sensory** or **afferent** neuron at the body's surface that communicates directly to a **motor** or **efferent** neuron that excites contractile cells.

In other types of jellyfish there exists the most complex form of the reflex arc: a three-neuron system. The sensory neurons no longer communicate directly with the motor neurons. Instead, an **intermediate** or **interneuron** acts as the go-between. Furthermore, these interneurons can create a network or **plexus** separating sensory and motor neurons.

In the case of man and other higher animals, a **brain** and **spinal cord** are formed by these interneuron networks: the **central nervous system.** (See Figure 14.)

The spinal cord contains (1) sensory pathways that convey neural information from the periphery to the brain, (2) motor pathways that send neural responses from the brain to the organs and tissues, and (3) interneurons.

The brain can be divided simply into two portions: the **hindbrain** and the **forebrain.** (See Figure 15.) The hindbrain includes the **brainstem,** which is involved in regulation of visceral functions like blood pressure and respiration. The other major part of the hindbrain

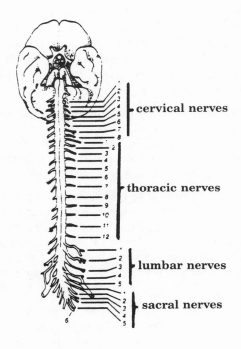

FIGURE 14 — **The central nervous system: the brain and spinal cord.** Note that the **peripheral nervous system** is made up of the spinal nerves and their branches outside of the spinal cord and is divided into two subsystems: the **neuromuscular (somatic)** and the **autonomic nervous system.**

118

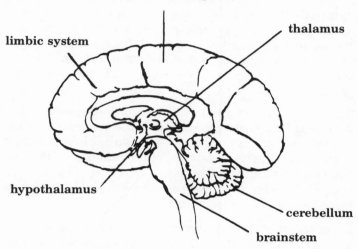

FIGURE 15 — **Important structures of the human brain.** A midsagittal section is shown (i.e., the brain is cut down the middle, from front to back).

is the **cerebellum.** The cerebellum functions in involuntary coordination of movements.

The forebrain is also commonly divided into two regions: the **diencephalon** and the **telencephalon.** The diencephalon includes the **thalamus**—which is a "relay station" for incoming sensory information—and the **hypothalamus**—which regulates the body temperature, water balance, fat and sugar metabolism, autonomic functions, and secretions of the endocrine glands.

The telencephalon portion of the forebrain contains the **cerebral hemispheres** (**cortex**), the conscious, thinking brain. It also contains the **subcortical structures**—the **limbic system** and **basal ganglia.** The limbic system and basal ganglia function in the regulation of emotional responses and in planning intentional movement, respectively.

Together, the sensory and motor neurons outside the spinal cord and brain make up the **peripheral nervous system,** which usually is divided into two components: the **somatic** or **neuromuscular system** and the **autonomic nervous system.** (See Figure 14.)

The neuromuscular system has been called the "voluntary" portion of the peripheral system, responding to the external environment by means of the skeletal muscles. (See Chapter 16.)

The autonomic nervous system is the involuntary or "vegetative" portion of the peripheral nervous system and innervates the glands and heart muscle as well as the smooth muscle found in the walls of the blood vessels and organs. The autonomic nervous system is further divided into two functional branches or divisions: the **sympathetic** (arousal responses) and the **parasympathetic** (nurturing response). (See Chapter 17.)

The next three chapters will examine how touch-oriented therapies affect neural function. Chapter 16 will examine the effects of somato-therapies on the neuromuscular system: muscle tone, posture, and movement; while Chapter 17 will cover the autonomic nervous system.

This chapter will explore the influences of somato-interventions on the brain and spinal cord: the central nervous system.

Somato-Techniques and the Central Nervous System

Recent clinical reports and research suggest that deep tactile stimulation through manipulation and acupuncture can help in rehabilitating patients with neurological disorders.

Gibbs (1984) reported the use of "deep muscle massage and acupuncture" along with biofeedback in the treatment of head injuries, strokes, and other neuromuscular disorders. He hypothesizes that the sensory stimulation induced by touch "alters the electrical activity" (e.g., brainwave patterns) in the central nervous system.

Deep pressure has also been tried in arousing patients out of coma. In one program, families of coma victims were taught to stimulate the patient's sensory system by applying deep pressure and movements to alternate limbs. This type of stimulation was continued for 11 to 14 hours a day (Phillips, 1983). According to Phillips, 92 percent of the patients were aroused from coma; of those, 35 percent resumed normal functioning.

In a study involving (osteopathic) craniosacral technique, a group of coma patients with long-standing spinal and brain damage were found to have "cranial rhythms" of 3 to 4 cycles per minute, which is about half the frequency for normal adults (Upledger and Vredevoogd, 1983). The amplitudes of the cranial rhythms were also about half the normal adult levels. The cranial rhythms were determined by palpation of the cranium and extremities as well as with a plethysmographic device. No conclusions were made concerning the possible use of craniosacral therapy for comatose patients.

Silverman (1973) conducted a study which lends some support to the notion that somato-therapy alters electrical brainwave activity (i.e., EEG's). EEG patterns (averaged evoked responses), eye movements, and a battery of biochemical tests were performed on 15 adult male subjects undergoing the Rolfing method of soft-tissue manipulation. The measurements were recorded before and after the manipulative interventions. Of interest was the finding that the post-test differences in EEG recordings suggested "an increased openness and receptivity" by the subjects to sensory stimulation when compared to their pre-test EEG recordings.

The exact nature of the physiological mechanism behind the findings cited above is not known. However, tactile stimulation to the sensory receptors in the skin, muscles, and other soft tissues appears to alter electrical activity in the brain. This change in neural activity seems to modify the overall "interpretation" of incoming sensory information by the central nervous system; and thus the motor responses to the organs, muscles, glands, and other tissues are altered. In other words, there seems to be a sensory or afferent loop that changes central neural processing and motor outflow when appropriately stimulated by somato-techniques.

Spinal Adjustments and Spinal Nerve Roots

A basic premise of both chiropractic and osteopathic approaches is that a "subluxation" of a vertebra will partially occlude the invertebral foramen and thereby interfere with the normal functioning of the spinal nerve root that passes through this opening. (See Chapters 6 and 7.)

There are thousands of case studies in chiropractic and osteopathic literature of cures for a variety of musculoskeletal and other physical ailments by means of spinal adjustments. There is also some preliminary evidence that supports the subluxation premise.

It has been proposed that spinal nerve roots are more likely to undergo "compression blockage" than are peripheral nerves (Sharpless, MacGraegor, and Luttges, 1975).

This position is supported by the work of osteopathic research (Korr, 1955). Korr found in a subluxated vertebral segment that the "anterior and lateral horn cells" were hypersensitive to stimulation, which in turn produced a rise in neural transmission rate. This increased firing rate of impulses was reported to alter functioning in organs and tissues, including vasoconstruction of blood vessels and increased muscle activity.

Further evidence comes from an experiment in which rabbits' vertebrae were manually subluxated. Later examination of tissue revealed that pathological damage had occurred in the subluxated segment (Cleveland, 1965).

Therapeutic Benefits

Most of the evidence concerning body therapy and higher neural function consists of clinical case studies and some preliminary experimental investigations. Yet there is reason to believe that touch-oriented methods are beneficial to the central nervous system function. Three main areas look especially promising:

1. The use of manipulative therapies and acupuncture in the rehabilitative treatment of neurological disorders such as head trauma and coma. Recent evidence suggests that brain functions (e.g., brainwave patterns) are affected by tactile procedures.
2. For spinal dysfunction involving the vertebral subluxation of nerve roots, spinal manipulation appears to be an appropriate treatment (e.g., for whiplash, headaches, and lower back strain).
3. Tactile stimulation of the sensory pathways may in turn alter how the brain modulates or interprets incoming sensory information.

The last area has implications for the treatment of learning disabilities: hyperactivity, autism, and mental retardation. For example, in one study a group of "brain injured" children were treated with the Rolfing manipulative method. Some of the children showed a marked improvement in cognitive, language, and social skills as well as the expected structural changes in movement and posture (Frazee, 1964).

REFERENCES

Cleveland, G.S. Researching the subluxation on the domestic rabbit. *Science Review of Chiropractic,* 1965, *1,* (4).

Frazee, J. Project Breakthrough success. *Foundation for Brain Injured Children Newsletter,* 1964, *1,* 1–2.

Gibbs, E. Neuro-kinesthetics. *Brain/Mind Bulletin,* 1984, *9*(8), 3.

Korr, I.M. Symposium of the functional implications of segmental facilitation. *Journal of the American Osteopathic Association,* 1955, *55*(1).

Nauta, W.H., and Feirtag, M. Organization of the brain. *Scientific American,* 1979, *241*(3), 88-111.

Phillips, R. Heavy stimulation, GSR, biofeedback, arouse patients from longterm coma. *Brain/Mind Bulletin,* 1983, *9*(1), 1–2.

Sharpless, S.K., MacGraegor, R.J., and Luttges, M.V. A pressure vessel model for nerve compression. *Journal for Neurological Sciences,* 1975, *24,* 299–304.

Silverman, J., et al. Stress, stimulus intensity control, and the Structural Integration technique. *Confinia Psychiatrica,* 1973, *16,* 201–219.

Upledger, J.E., and Vredevoogd, J.D. *Craniosacral Therapy.* Chicago: Eastland Press, 1983.

. . . the motor act is the cradle of the mind.
— *C.S. Sherrington*

CHAPTER 16
MUSCLE TONE, POSTURE, AND MOVEMENT

Overview

The skeletal or striated muscles, along with the connective-tissue network, are responsible for posture, movement, and structural shape of the body. (See also Chapter 14.) The skeletal muscles are richly innervated by sensory and motor nerve fibers and therefore are regulated by the nervous system, hence the name **neuromuscular system.**

The neuromuscular system has certain unique properties that permit the carrying out of its functions (Chusid, 1976):

1. **Contractility:** the capacity to contract or shorten is found in all cells, but muscle tissue is specialized in this function.
2. **Elasticity:** depending on the pattern of nerve impulses, muscles will shorten or lengthen.
3. **Extensibility:** muscle has the ability to lengthen when stretched.
4. **Irritability:** the capacity to respond to different forms of stimulation (e.g., touch, electrical, heat, etc.) by either contracting or lengthening.

Muscle tissue's property of irritability, to respond to different forms of tactile stimulation, is the underlying basis for somato-therapies' effects on muscle tone, posture, and voluntary movement.

Muscle Tone and Spinal Reflexes

Muscle tone refers to the constant state of contraction for a muscle in a given postural position (e.g., sitting, lying down, or standing). As shall be examined below, the amount of muscle tone in a given muscle is primarily dependent on the neural transmission from the spinal cord and brain.

It is known that sensory receptors or "sensors" within the myofascial tissues (i.e., muscle, fascia, ligaments, and tendons) react to mechanical stretching and shortening (Shepherd, 1983). There are two types of sensors involved: (1) the **muscle spindles** and (2) the **Golgi tendon organs.**

Muscle spindles are encapsulated structures located throughout the skeletal musculature. Because of their enclosed fusiform shape, they are referred to as **intrafusal** muscle fibers and are located within and parallel to the larger **extrafusal** muscle fibers that make up the contractile portion of the muscle. (See Figure 16.) (The muscle spindle's function in maintaining posture will be discussed in the next section.)

When the muscle is suddenly stretched, the encapsulated muscle spindles are also stretched. This stretching stimulates or "loads" the muscle spindle, which then sends nerve impulses to motor neurons (alpha) in the spinal cord, instructing the muscle to contract (i.e., increase its tone). (See Figure 16.) This contracting of a muscle, or group of muscles, that follows a quick stretching is called the **stretch reflex.** Note that the **antagonistic muscles,** having the opposite movement function, will lengthen.

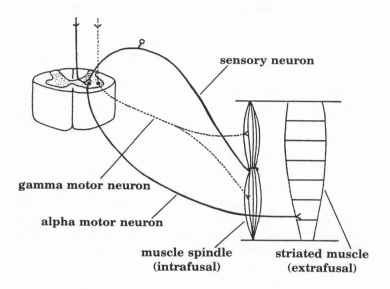

sensory neuron

gamma motor neuron

alpha motor neuron

**muscle spindle
(intrafusal)**

**striated muscle
(extrafusal)**

FIGURE 16 — **Gamma and alpha motor neuron systems.** A gamma neuron is shown innervating a muscle spindle, while the alpha motor neuron innervates a larger, striated muscle. Note that the muscle spindle and striated muscle have a parallel alignment. A sensory fiber from the muscle spindle synapses in the spinal cord onto an alpha motor neuron. When the muscle spindle is "loaded" (stretched), this sensory fiber increases its firing rate, thereby increasing muscle tone; when the muscle spindle is "unloaded" (shortened), the muscle tone is decreased. Thus, the muscle spindle has been described as the "sensing element" of the neuromuscular system, keeping the larger skeletal muscles at a relatively constant length under different amounts of tension.

If the muscle is mechanically shortened (e.g., tactile pressure to the belly of the muscle), the muscle spindle is shortened or "unloaded," decreasing its firing rate to motor neurons in the spinal cord. Thus the muscle is lengthened, and muscle tone is reduced. In this case the antagonistic muscles will be shortened. Such a procedure is frequently utilized in massage and soft-tissue manipulation when a certain muscle is "hypertoned" and needs to be relaxed.

The Golgi tendon organs, like the muscle spindles, are encapsulated structures. But unlike the muscle spindles, they are located in the collagenous fibers of tendons, ligaments, and fascial sheaths—usually near the bony insertions (Carpenter and Sutin, 1983). The Golgi tendon organs have sensory nerve endings that terminate within minute bundles of collagen fibers. Because they are in "series" with the tendon and fascial fibers, they primarily respond to tension.

When, for instance, the tendon is slowly and actively stretched (e.g., deep pressure), the Golgi tendon organs increase their firing rate. These impulses are sent to the spinal cord and inhibit alpha motor neurons and muscle tone. (See Figure 17.) At the same time, the tone of the antagonistic muscles is increased.

Soft-tissue methods utilize the Golgi tendon organs and the associated spinal reflexes to lengthen muscles by actively stretching the fascial sheaths and applying deep pressure to tendon insertions. Similarly, the slow stretching produced by Hatha yoga postures also stimulates Golgi-tendon reflex arcs. Note that a slow, steady rise in stretch force will relax the muscle tone, while a

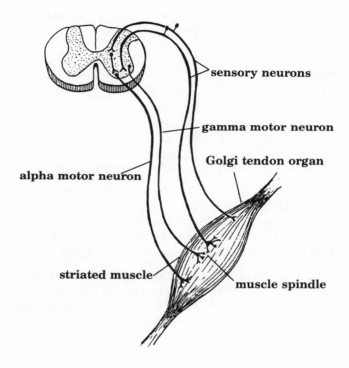

FIGURE 17 — **Golgi tendon organ.** Slow and active stretching of a muscle tendon will increase the Golgi tendon organ's firing rate. These impulses are sent to the spinal cord, where they inhibit alpha motor neurons and relax muscle tone. Soft-tissue manipulation and Hatha yoga both utilize the Golgi tendon reflex arc.

quick rise in stretch force will elicit a shortening of the muscle through the stretch reflex.

Posture

The effects of somato-procedures appear to have more than just local consequences to the muscle under stimulation. Entire postural patterns of muscle tone have been reported to be altered by somato-therapies. These clinical observations suggest that muscle tone and posture are not regulated solely by spinal reflexes.

In fact, it is known that higher brain centers are involved in the modulation of posture and associated muscle tone as well as movement. The brain regions include the brainstem, cerebellum, basal ganglia, thalamus, and cerebral cortex. (See Figure 18.)

While the **alpha motor neurons** control the contraction of the large extrafusal muscle fibers which produce active movement, it is the **gamma motor neurons** that innervate the muscle spindles (intrafusal fibers). (See Figure 16.)

The muscle spindles can be described as the "sensing element" of the neuromuscular system. That is, the muscle spindles register differences in length between themselves and the larger extrafusal muscle fibers that surround them. There are two types of muscle spindles: "dynamic" and "static." Dynamic muscle spindles respond to changes in muscle length produced by stretching or compression. Static muscle spindles respond to changes in the tensional force placed on the muscle (e.g., changes in the gravitational force as the body shifts).

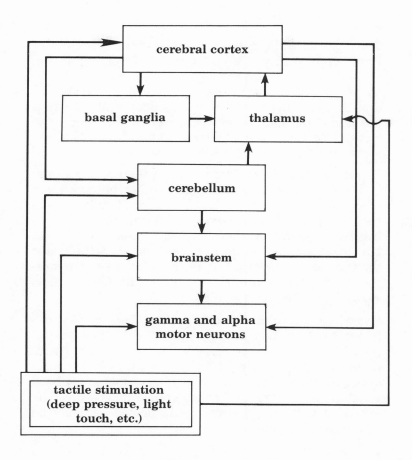

FIGURE 18 — **Higher neural centers' control of muscle tone, posture, and movement and the influences of tactile stimulation on this regulation.**

Thus, the gamma motor neurons and muscle spindles function primarily at an unconscious level, regulating muscle tone, postures, and fine adjustments that form the "background" for active movement produced by the alpha motor neurons. Recent research indicates that the alpha and gamma systems are "co-activated," the gamma system being activated only when there is some tension or "load" placed on the muscle.

Higher centers in the brain can influence the alpha and gamma motor neurons through descending nerve tracts that travel down the spinal cord. The higher centers may have either an **excitatory** (facilitatory) or an **inhibitory** effect on these two motor neuron systems. For example, any given excitatory input would have the end result of increasing muscle tone to certain muscle groups (e.g., flexors), while an inhibitory input would have the opposite result.

Experimental animal studies support the idea that different types of tactile stimulation will affect overall muscle tone and hence posture. The tactile sensory information is sent to the brain, where after "processing," output is sent to the alpha and gamma motor neurons, which in turn determine muscle tone and posture. The effects of various types of tactile procedures may be summarized as follows:

1. Gentle stroking of the back reduced shivering in cats and was interpreted as an inhibition of the gamma motor neuron system (von Euler and Soderberg, 1958). Such light touch also produced autonomic changes, therefore indicating involvement of higher brain centers. (See Chapter 17.)
2. Slow, deep pressure to the soft tissues of cats was

associated with a reduction in electromylographic activity in muscles, indicating a relaxation of muscle tone (Johansson, 1962).

3. Pinching, sudden deep tactile pressure, and other painful somato-procedures are known to induce a general contraction of the musculature, particularly in muscles used in flexion (Eble, 1960; Jones, 1965).

That somato-intervention can evoke systemic changes in neuromuscular activity is given further support through numerous studies involving the use of photographs and radiographs. Investigators have demonstrated changes in posture and musculoskeletal alignment for several somato-therapeutic techniques: Rolfing (Solit, 1962); Alexander technique (Jones, 1965); chiropractic spinal manipulation (Palmer, 1938); and osteopathic craniosacral therapy (Greenman, 1970).

Somato-Techniques and Movement

Sherrington (1906) was the first to distinguish the differences between "active" voluntary movement and "passive" reflexive movement in terms of how they are regulated by the nervous system. Yet it is difficult to separate the "unconscious" movements involving postural adjustments from the larger, voluntary, "conscious" movements of walking, reaching, sitting down, and so forth.

In reality, voluntary movement is performed on a background of postural, spinal reflexes that keep the body in an upright and balanced relationship to the gravitational field (see preceding sections).

Complex movements appear to be based on rhythmic, sequential patterns of neuromuscular activity. Such "rhythm generators" have been found in the spines of dogs for walking and scratching (Evarts, 1979). The cerebral cortex and other higher centers can then modify the specifics of the movement pattern being generated.

The question that will be explored here is whether tactile intervention can affect complex movements by altering the pattern of neural outflow to the muscles.

In a study of human subjects involving multiple-image photography, Jones (1965) reported that different basic movements can be modified by the application of gentle directional pressure to the body, by using the Alexander technique. (See Chapter 8.) The movements examined were: lying down to sitting up, sitting to standing, leaning forward to sitting erectly, and walking.

A subject's "habitual" movement patterns were first filmed as a pre-test or control. This was then followed by the experimental or "guided" procedures by the experimenter and another post-test filming.

The subjects filmed in the experimental condition showed the trajectory of the head to be higher and the arch of the movements to be smoother and more regular. The movement pattern was "characteristically" altered "when the relation of head and trunk" had been modified by the guided procedures. The most dramatic result obtained was in the sitting to standing movement.

Jones interpreted the results as a facilitation of the "righting reflexes" of the head and neck that return the body to a normal upright posture in relation to gravity. Jones proposed that these postural, righting reflexes were normally masked by habitual, voluntary activity or "attitudinal reflexes"—movement that is habitually used to obtain a special purpose (e.g., reaching for an object, lookup upward, etc.):

> In the attitudinal reflexes, the head is drawn into a fixed position and tonus (tone) is redistributed in the trunk and limbs. In righting reflexes, again under the influence of the head, normal distribution of the tonus is restored. . . . The procedures employed in the experimental movements by releasing the head from its habitual attitude, facilitate the righting reflexes and bring the subject into a different orientation to the gravitational field. (Jones, 1965, p. 210)

Jones considered the attitudinal reflexes under the control of the cerebral cortex, while the antigravity righting reflexes were maintained at the subcortical and spinal levels (Jones, 1963, 1965).

Thus the smoother, efficient movements observed under the guided-experimental condition are apparently due to an inhibition of higher conscious (cortical) centers of the brain. This inhibition in turn allows the spinal and subcortical postural reflexes and rhythmic movement patterns to function freely.

Hunt and Massey (1977) conducted an electromyographic (EMG) analysis concerning the effects of the

Rolfing method on movement. (Electromyographic re-cordings measure the electrical activity in muscles.)

A control and an experimental group each containing 24 subjects all performed six activities: lying, throw-ing, lifting, jogging, stepping up onto a stool, and ka-rate chop. The subjects were matched for age, birth de-fects, injuries, weight, and height. Telemetry elec-tromyographic recordings were taken from 16 separate muscles as a pre-test. The experimental group under-went ten sessions of the Rolfing method over a time of five weeks. Following the five-week period, the experi-mental and control groups were again given a post-test evaluation.

Hunt and Massey found that post-tests for the experi-mental group showed a decrease in EMG activity in antagonist muscles. They interpreted this finding as representing more efficient movement patterns with less "joint excursion" and compression. The control's post-tests, in contrast to the experimental group's, showed more electrical activity in both antagonistic and agonist muscles, suggesting that more energy was expended in carrying out the test movements.

They further reported that the post-tests of the experi-mental group exhibited the most improvement in the action of deeper, intrinsic muscles located proximally (i.e., nearer) to the joints.

Similar to Jones' position and findings with the Alex-ander technique, Hunt and Massey concluded that the Rolfing treatments altered the neural control of move-ment in the direction of subcortical and spinal levels, away from the conscious cortical influence.

Both of the above-cited research studies indicate that certain body procedures lead to the inhibition of "conscious" control over repetitive habitual movements, allowing the more "unconscious," spinal and subcortical levels of movement patterns to dominate.

Therapeutic Benefits

The neuromuscular system is affected by somatotherapies on three different levels: individual muscle tone, postural patterns, and voluntary movement.

1. **First level:** Tactile stimulation through massage, pressure, and manipulation excites sensors within the individual muscles, fascial sheaths, and tendons, which induces spinal reflex arcs. These reflexes in turn increase or decrease the state of muscle contraction or tone in the stimulated muscle as well as in its antagonists.

   Such procedures are utilized extensively in the treatment of athletic injuries as well as for the management of muscular "tension" or "stress." For example, "muscle cramps" commonly experienced by athletes are reduced or eliminated by stretching the muscle to its full length and holding the stretch for approximately two minutes (deVries, 1966).

2. **Second level:** Certain techniques of body therapy (e.g., Rolfing, Alexander technique, chiropractic, and osteopathy) have been shown to produce remarkable changes in individual postural patterns, indicating an overall integration of neuromuscular balance.

3. **Third level:** Experimental, controlled studies have reported evidence that both the Alexander

technique and the Rolfing method alter movement patterns towards more efficient use of muscular energy.

The last two levels suggest a wide range of benefits, particularly with the treatment of neuromuscular disorders: cerebral palsy, stroke, and nerve "compression syndromes." (See Chapters 14 and 15.) Athletic injuries as well as athletic performances are also areas that have great potential.

A final potential of therapeutic use concerns prevention of neuromuscular injuries and dysfunctions. Though to date little research has been done, prevention may turn out to be the most significant benefit.

REFERENCES

Carpenter, M.B., and Sutin, J. *Human Neuroanatomy.* Baltimore/London: Williams and Wilkins, 1983.

Chusid, J.G. *Correlative Neuroanatomy and Functional Neurology.* Los Altos, CA: Lange Medical Publications, 1976.

deVries, H.A. Quantitative electromyographic investigation of the spasm theory of muscle pain. *American Journal of Physical Medicine,* 1966, *45,* 119–134.

Eble, J.N. Patterns of response of the paravertebral musculature to visceral stimuli. *Americal Journal of Physiology,* 1960, *198,* 429–433.

Evarts, E.V. Brain mechanisms of movement. *Scientific American,* 1979, *241* (3), 164–179.

Greenman, P.E. Roentgen findings in the craniosacral mechanism. *Journal of the American Osteopathic Association,* 1970, *70,* 24–35.

Hunt, V.V., and Massey, W. *A Study of Structural Integration from Neuromuscular, Energy Field, and Emotional Approaches.* Boulder, Colorado: Rolf Institute, 1977.

Johansson, B. Circulatory response to stimulation of somatic afferents. *Acta Physiologica Scandinavica,* 1962, *62* (Supplementum 198), 1–91.

Jones, F.P. The influence of postural set on pattern movement in man. *International Journal of Neurology,* 1963, *4,* 60–71.

Jones, F.P. Method for changing stereotyped response patterns by the inhibition of certain postural sets. *Psychological Review,* 1965, *72,* 196–214.

Palmer, B.J. *Precise, Posture Constant Spinograph Comparative Graphs.* Davenport, Iowa: Palmer School of Chiropractic, 1938.

Shepherd, G.M. *Neurobiology.* New York/Oxford: Oxford University Press, 1983.

Sherrington, C.S. *The Integrative Action of the Nervous System.* New York: Charles Scribner's Sons, 1906.

Solit, M. A study in structural dynamics. *Journal of the American Osteopathic Association,* 1962, *62,* 30–40.

Von Euler, C., and Soderberg, V. Co-ordinated changes in temperature thresholds for thermoregulatory reflexes. *Acta Physiologica Scandinavica,* 1958, *42,* 112–129.

... there is a basis for arguing that autonomic changes do occur when this myofascial "web" is appropriately altered towards more balanced functioning [through manipulation]. It would be useful to measure these autonomic changes. ...

— *Peter A. Levine*

Thus, the evaluation of heart rate patterns [an autonomic measure], ... may function as a diagnostic window to the brain.

— *Stephen W. Porges*

CHAPTER 17
BALANCE OF THE AUTONOMIC
NERVOUS SYSTEM

Overview

By the early 20th century, the concept of disease being a consequence of imbalance between two complementary, antagonistic forces appeared in Western science with the description of the autonomic nervous system and its two anatomical and functional branches: **parasympathetic (PNS)** and **sympathetic (SNS).**

Langley (1921) coined the term **autonomic,** meaning the "self-governing" portion of the peripheral nervous system that innervates the smooth muscle of the heart, blood vessels, glands, and other viscera. This was contrasted to the "voluntary" or **somatic** part of the peripheral nervous system that supplies motor control to the voluntary skeletal muscles. (See also Chapter 16.) The distinction between autonomic and voluntary motor systems is now considered somewhat artificial in that both are integrated and modulated by higher neural centers including the hypothalamus, portions of the limbic system, and the brainstem (Nauta and Feirtag, 1979).

Eppinger and Hess (1917) proposed an early autonomic theory relating specific nervous disorders to pathological imbalances between the parasympathetic and sympathetic divisions.

Cannon (1932) hypothesized that the consistency or "homeostasis" of the internal environment was controlled by the outflow of the two autonomic branches.

147

The sympathetic portion with its innervation of the adrenal medulla is involved in arousal or emergency responses. The SNS remains active at all times (as does the parasympathetic), but can increase its peripheral outflow as a unit under conditions of mobilization— Cannon's "fight-flight" response. Under such mobilization, the heart rate is accelerated, blood pressure increases; blood flow is shifted from the skin and internal organs to the skeletal muscles; blood sugar rises; blood adrenalin rises; and airway passages and pupils dilate (Ganong, 1977).

In global terms, Cannon saw sympathetic outflow concerned with catabolic functions that mobilized the body, while parasympathetic outflow usually involved the anabolic functions of nurturing and rebuilding. Yet recent research indicates a more complex picture. A given target organ appears quite specific in its response to both sympathetic and parasympathetic stimulation (Goodman and Gillman, 1980). (See Table 3.)

Parasympathetic outflow is largely through the parasympathetic fibers of the **vagus** nerve (often simply termed "vagal outflow"). Its activities include an increase in gastrointestinal, hepatic, and pancreatic secretions; an increase in gastrointestinal movements; a decrease in heart rate; an increase of blood to the gut out of the skeletal muscles; and constriction of air-way passages (Ganong, 1977).

The two divisions usually work as antagonists: if one branch increases a given process (e.g., heart rate), the other branch is typically inhibitive (Higgins, et al., 1973). Yet there are instances when SNS and PNS work synergistically (e.g., salivation) and cases when only

Target Organ	Parasympathetic Function	Sympathetic Function
Eye	stimulates ciliary muscle and sphincter pupillae—pupillary constriction to light and during accomodation	stimulates dilator pupillae and possibly radial fibers of ciliary muscle—pupillary dilatation
Lacrimal, nasal, palatine, and salivary glands	stimulates secretory cells—serous and mucous secretions	no important effect
Heart	inhibits intrinsic cardiac activity— heart rate slows	stimulates intrinsic cardiac activity— heart rate increases
Tracheobronchial tree	stimulates secretory cells and smooth muscle—serous and mucous secretions, narrowing of bronchioles	inhibits smooth muscle —relaxation of bronchioles
Alimentary canal	stimulates secretory cells and smooth muscle—digestive secretions, peristalsis, evacuation	inhibits smooth muscle —decreases peristalsis
Liver and pancreas	stimulates pancreatic cells (effect on liver unknown)	no important effect
Adrenal medulla	no effect	stimulates secretory cells—secretion of epinephrine
Urinary bladder	stimulates smooth muscle (detrusor)— emptying of bladder	no effect on emptying; may activate internal sphincter during ejaculation
Genital organs	uncertain and variable; may stimulate smooth muscle and glands; vascular dilatation	uncertain and variable; may stimulate vaso-constriction

TABLE 3 — **Summary of autonomic functions.** In general the sympathetic branch is concerned with arousal and mobilization of the body; the parasympathetic branch, in contrast, is involved in nurturing and rebuilding processes. The two divisions usually work as antagonists, but there are exceptions.

149

one division is involved (e.g., control of the peripheral vasculature by the sympathetics).

According to Gellhorn's (1957) theory of autonomic balance, the two autonomic components have a general antagonistic relationship. His **law of reciprocal innervation** states that the "excitation" of one autonomic branch induces a simultaneous "inhibition" of the other branch. Gellhorn also described a **rebound phenomenon** that immediately follows the transient stimulation of one of the divisions. This rebound principle involves a "waning" of activity in the stimulated division and a "waxing" of response in the nonstimulated branch.

Gellhorn (1967) further reported a condition of **autonomic tuning** in which the activity of one branch was tuned up, while the output of the other branch was dampened during prolonged stimulation of the former (e.g., experimentally induced stress). Tuning implies a permanent change in the level of autonomic output, and thus the expected rebound phenomenon is lost. For example, an animal whose hypothalamus is stimulated electrically to induce a constant state of sympathetic activation would eventually show a permanent increase in SNS activity and reduction in PNS, thereby becoming "sympathetically tuned."

A comparison can be made between the yin-yang concept of balance from ancient Chinese medicine and modern theories of autonomic balance. (See Chapter 1.)

Stated simply, overactivity of the sympathetic branch ("sympathetic tuning"), a chronic arousal response, has a striking overall similarity to the hyperactive characteristics of "excess yang" diseases. In turn, chronic overactivity of the parasympathetic branch ("parasympathetic tuning") appears to parallel the hypo-mobility of fatigue ailments found in "excess yin" patterns.

Whether the parallels between the two primordial forces found in traditional Chinese medicine and the modern construct of a dynamic balance between the two autonomic divisions will hold under closer examination is open to question. Still, the comparison is appealing.

Contemporary Body Therapies and Autonomic Balance

While modern theories of the autonomic nervous system were being developed, practitioners of musculoskeletal manipulation began concurrently to relate the consequences of their therapeutic procedures to alterations in autonomic function. Clinically, they observed that as structural deficiencies and asymmetries in musculoskeletal structure became reorganized or "balanced," a parallel reorganization in the nervous system appeared to follow.

From these clinical reports, certain manipulative procedures became associated with an increase or decrease in sympathetic or parasympathetic output. Techniques that are considered to produce a sympathetic response are termed **sympathicotonic,** while manipulations thought to evoke a vagal (parasympathetic) response are called **vagotonic.**

Of particular interest are the somato-therapies involving soft tissue and spinal manipulations—that is, techniques that work on the body's bony skeleton and connective tissues (fascia, muscle, and the tendonous insertions). Methods that make reference to autonomic integration as a consequence of such interventions include the Rolfing technique, osteopathic craniosacral therapy, chiropractic spinal manipulation, and Reichian therapy.

Upledger (1983) described one of the primary benefits of osteophatic craniosacral therapy as "the restoration of autonomic flexibility." (See Chapter 6.)

A similar position is made for chiropractic spinal manipulation and enhancement of autonomic activity (Homewood, 1977). (See Chapter 7.)

Similarly, Reich (1973) stated that the goal of his vegetotherapy was, in part, to restore autonomic function, a balance between two biological poles, "expansion" (i.e., parasympathetic) and contraction (i.e., sympathetic). (See Chapter 10.)

Rolf (1977), the developer of the Rolfing method, was influenced by early osteopathic medicine which emphasized the role of fascial connective tissue in both structural and physiological function. Rolf proposed that structural balance of the "myofascial component" is necessary for optimal autonomic and higher neural function. For Rolf, the method for approaching neural-autonomic balance was through the structural reorganization of the "myofascial web." (See Chapter 9.)

Research Concerning Tactile Interventions and Autonomic Reflexes

The autonomic nervous system is known to have reflex pathways similar to the muscle-tone reflexes described in Chapter 16. Autonomic reflexes involve sensory fibers from both visceral organs and somatic structures. Autonomic reflexes, like those innervating the skeletal muscles, can be controlled at the level of the spinal cord or can be influenced by higher neural centers.

As previously mentioned, portions of the brainstem, hypothalamus, limbic system, and the cerebral cortex modulate autonomic functions. The **hypothalamus,** however, is the "hub" for autonomic regulation, receiving sensory input from various sources and sending out motor information through the sympathetic and parasympathetic branches to the organs and tissues in the periphery (MacLean, 1955). The hypothalamus also plays an integral role in regulating the endocrine system and assists in the maintaining of muscle tone and posture.

The observations made by somato-therapists that a given tactile manipulation produces either a vagotonic or a sympathicotonic response is supported by animal and human studies involving tactile stimulation and autonomic reflexes.

Folkow (1962) found that abdominal surgical manipulations performed on humans induced a "vagal reflex" involving a decrease in blood pressure and heart rate (i.e., an increase in parasympathetic response). He also was able to elicit an identical vagal reflex by electrical stimulation of visceral sensory fibers. Johansson (1962) reported similar vagotonic effects involving a decrease in blood pressure (i.e., "depressor reflex") when deep tactile pressure was applied to certain skeletal muscles of cats.

Johansson (1962) also found that pinching the muscle and skin or applying friction to the skin of cats evoked a sympathicotonic response involving an increase of blood pressure (i.e., "pressor reflex").

Different patterns of electrical stimulation to the skin of freely moving cats had marked effects on EEG (i.e., brain waves) as well as EMG (i.e., electrical activity) in muscles (Pompeiano and Swett, 1962). Slow patterns of stimulation produced a synchronization of the EEG, behavioral sleep symptoms, and a reduction in EMG activity—indicating a predominance of parasympathetic response. Higher rates of stimulation induced an "arousal" EEG pattern and an increase in EMG activity; thus, higher frequencies of stimulation appeared to evoke a sympathicotonic response.

Porter, Marshall, and Porges (1984) reported that in infants undergoing circumcision, heart rate increased and heart-rate variability decreased. They concluded that the painful stimulation of circumcision produced a transient drop in parasympathetic activity (i.e., vagal tone) as well as a possible increase in sympathetic activity.

In summary, the studies suggest that slow, deep manipulative pressure to the muscles or abdominal viscera produce parasympathetic reflex responses that include a decrease in blood pressure and heart rate, a synchronizing of EEG's, and a decrease in baseline EMG activity. Light touch to the skin appears to induce a similar vagotonic response. In contrast, painful touch to the skin or musculature induces an arousal, or sympathicotonic response, that includes an increase in blood pressure and heart rate, an arousal EEG pattern, and an increase in EMG activity. Finally, various rates or patterns of stimulation appear to evoke different autonomic responses.

Muscular Core-Sleeve Types and Autonomic Function

Recently, the author completed a pilot study that explored the effects of certain soft-tissue manipulations on parasympathetic function. Musculoskeletal structure was also compared to autonomic responses (Cottingham and Porges, 1984).

Parasympathetic activity was determined by measuring the variations in the heart pattern that are associated with normal breathing. This autonomic index was developed by Porges (1983) and termed "vagal tone."

Photographs were also taken of each subject. From the photographs, an independent rater placed the subjects in one of four possible groupings according to **core-sleeve** muscular patterns. Silverman (1973) first described this method by which subjects were classified by the relative muscle tone of the deeper, intrinsic "core" muscles to the outer, extrinsic "sleeve" muscles. Four groupings are commonly made (see Figure 19):

1. A "balance" between the core and sleeve musculature
2. A hypertoned "hard" core and a hypotoned or "soft" sleeve
3. A "soft" core and a "hard" sleeve
4. A "mixed" or confused core-sleeve relationship

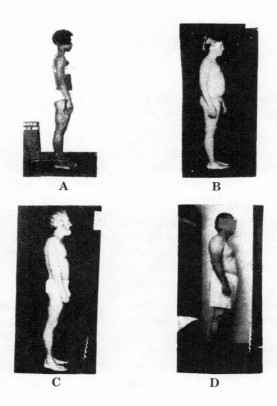

FIGURE 19 — **The four core-sleeve groupings.** This classification is determined by the relative muscle tone of the deeper,
intrinsic core muscles to the outer, extrinsic sleeve muscles: (A)
"balanced" core-sleeve, (B) hypertoned or "hard" core and
hypotoned or "soft" sleeve, (C) "soft" core and "hard" sleeve, and
(D) "mixed" or confused core-sleeve relationship.

Four adult male subjects each received three procedures: two "vagotonic" and one "sympathicotonic":

1. Pressure with the hands to the costal and solar plexus regions (vagotonic)
2. Pelvic lift: the pelvis being turned under and back with gentle manipulative assistance (vagotonic)
3. Deep pressure with fingers to the plantar surface of the foot (sympathicotonic)

EKG and heart rate were also recorded.

The results supported the findings cited in the previous section. Three of the four subjects showed increases in parasympathetic activity during the administration of a hypothesized vagotonic procedure (pelvic lift). This was immediately followed by a "rebound" decrease in PNS response upon termination of the manipulation. (The subjects did not exhibit a noticeable shift in parasympathetic activity during the sympathicotonic manipulation.)

When subjects' autonomic responses were compared to their core-sleeve muscular classifications, individual differences were found. For example, the subject with the highest levels of PNS activity and the most flexibility (i.e., variability in response) was also rated as a "balanced" core-sleeve type. In sharp contrast, the subject with the lowest levels of parasympathetic activity and least flexibility of response was classified as a "mixed" core-sleeve pattern. These preliminary results suggest that optimal flexibility in autonomic response may be reflected in balanced musculoskeletal patterns. (See Figure 20.)

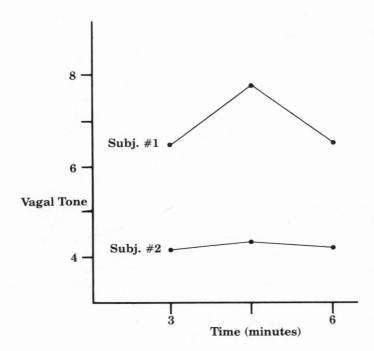

FIGURE 20 — **A vagotonic manipulation (pelvic lift) and
individual differences in autonomic response.** Subject #1
showed a large degree of "flexibility" in autonomic response
(vagal tone) and was rated as a "balanced" core-sleeve type.
Subject #2, on the other hand, exhibited very low autonomic
flexibility in terms of vagal tone and was rated as a "mixed"
core-sleeve type. The pilot study data suggested that optimal
autonomic flexibility may be correlated with a balanced musculoskeletal pattern.

Caution should be taken in interpreting data from such a small sample size; tentative inferences can be made at best. At the time of this writing, a full-scale investigation is under way.

Therapeutic Benefits

There is a growing body of literature which relates many diseases and behavioral problems to autonomic dysfunctions (Haynes, 1958; Gellhorn, 1967; Pelletier, 1977). Disorders considered to be caused, in part, by imbalances in autonomic response include high blood pressure, headaches, ulcers, asthma, colitis, psoriasis, hyperactivity, and autism. According to these theories, autonomic balance is a central concept in maintaining health and in prevention of disease.

There are also literally hundreds of case studies from the somato-therapeutic literature that report cures for the above and other disorders by means of "discharging," "balancing," and "increasing the flexibility" of autonomic function.

Preliminary evidence gives support to these theories and case studies. Somato-interventions can elicit transient vagotonic and sympathicotonic responses. The direction of the response seems to depend on two factors:

1. The type of tactile procedure being employed
2. The specific autonomic state of the individual (i.e., is he "sympathetically tuned" or "parasympathetically" biased)

The second factor, individual differences in autonomic status, appears to be crucial in determining the type of response that a given manipulation will induce. An illustration from the author's clinical practice is a client suffering from an acute "asthma attack." Presumably he is parasympathetically "tuned" (i.e., PNS constricts the airway passages). If a sympathicotonic procedure is administered, a PNS response may initially occur, producing further constriction of the airways, which, however, is then followed by a longer "rebound" rise in SNS activity and an opening of the airways.

Finally, individual differences in musculoskeletal structure like "core-sleeve" balance may also be intricately related to autonomic balance.

Do body therapies produce permanent or long-term autonomic changes? Although the case studies and anecdotal reports give strong support for such a contention, the answer is not known in terms of controlled clinical studies. This provocative question awaits further research.

REFERENCES

Cannon, W.B. *The Wisdom of the Body.* New York: Norton, 1932.

Cottingham, J.T., and Porges, S.W. The effects of soft manipulation on transient autonomic function. Unpublished manuscript, 1984.

Eppinger, H., and Hess, L. *Die Vegotonie.* Berlin, 1910 (Translation) *Vegatonia.* New York: Nervous and Mental Disease Publishing Co., 1917.

Folkow, B., et al. Cardiovascular reactions during abdominal surgery. *Annals of Surgery,* 1962, *156,* 905–913.

Ganong, W.F. *Review of Medical Physiology.* Los Altos, CA: Lange Medical Publications, 1977.

Gellhorn, E. *Autonomic Imbalance and the Hypothalamus.* Minneapolis: University of Minnesota Press, 1957.

Gellhorn, E. *Principles of Autonomic-Somatic Integrations: Physiological Basis and Psychological and Clinical Implications.* Minneapolis: University of Minnesota Press, 1967.

Goodman, L.S., and Gillman, A. (Eds.) *The Pharmacological Basis of Therapeutics.* New York: Macmillan, 1980.

Haynes, B. *Autonomic Dyspraxia.* London: H.K. Lewis, 1958.

Higgins, C.B., et al. Parasympathetic control of the heart. *Pharmacological Review,* 1973, *19,* 119–155.

Homewood, A.E. *The Neurodynamics of the Vertebral Subluxation.* St. Petersburg, Florida: Valkyrie Press Inc., 1977.

Johansson, B. Circulatory response to stimulation of somatic afferents. *Acta Physiologica Scandinavica,* 1962, *62,* (Supplementum 198), 1–91.

Langley, J.N. *The Autonomic Nervous System* (Vol. 1). Cambridge: Heffer and Sons, 1921.

MacLean, P.D. The limbic system ("visceral brain") and emotional behavior. *Arch. Neural. and Psychiat.*, 1955, *73*, 130–134.

Nauta, W.H., and Feirtag, M.J. Organization of the brain. *Scientific American,* 1979, *241* (3), 88–111.

Pelletier, K.R. *Mind as Healer, Mind as Slayer.* New York: Dell Publishing Co., Inc., 1977.

Pompeiano, O., and Swett, J.E. EEG and behavioral manifestations of sleep induced by cutaneous nerve stimulation in normal cats. *Arch. Ital. Biol.,* 1962, *100,* 311–342.

Porges, S.W. Heart rate patterns in neonates: a potential diagnostic window to the brain. In T. Field and A. Sostek (Eds.), *Infants Born at Risk.* New York: Grune and Stratton, Inc., 1983.

Porter, F., Marshall, R. and Porges, S.W. (in preparation) Vagal shifts during neonatal circumcision, 1984.

Reich, W. *The Function of Orgasm.* New York: Farrar, Straus, and Giroux, 1973.

Rolf, I.P. *Rolfing: the Integration of Human Structures.* Santa Monica, CA: Dennis-Landman Publishers, 1977.

Silverman, J., et al. Stress, stimulus intensity control, and the Structural Integration technique. *Confinia Psychiatrica,* 1973, *16,* 201–219.

Upledger, J.E., and Vredevoogd, J.D. *Craniosacral Therapy.* Chicago: Eastland Press, 1983.

The endorphins . . . are the morphine within.

— *Avram Goldstein*

CHAPTER 18
PAIN AND THE ENDOGENOUS
OPIATE SYSTEM

Overview

One of the most commonly reported effects of the somato-therapies is the reduction of pain. Extensive research has focused on the role that "acupuncture loci" and "trigger points" play in pain reduction.

It should be noted that many acupuncture points are identical to pressure points described in other body therapies (Melzack, Stillwell, and Fox, 1977). A number of the sites lie on the skin above major nerve trunks (Chu, Yeh, and Wood, 1979). A study by Becker (1976) found the electrical resistance of the cutaneous tissue above an acupuncture point to be significantly less than the adjacent region. The fascial layers of connective tissue have also been implicated (Oschman, 1981). (See also Chapters 1 and 14.)

Two theories have been proposed to account for the pain-relieving or **analgesic** properties that both direct pressure and indirect stimulation with needles produce. The **gate control theory** of pain involves the inhibition of sensory nerve fibers carrying pain information by other non-pain fibers. The **endogenous opiate theory** of pain proposes an "intrinsic analgesic system."

The Gate Control Theory of Pain

The gate control theory proposes that certain types of tactile pressure stimulate the larger sensory or afferent nerve fibers (A beta) located in the skin and muscle tissues. These high-velocity afferents, which respond to pressure and touch, connect (i.e., synapse) with inhibitory interneurons in the spinal cord. These inhibitory interneurons in turn block the transmission of neural impulses to the ascending, secondary pain fibers located in the spinal cord and thus create a "closed gate" condition. (See Figure 21.)

When, however, only the small, low-velocity sensory pain fibers (C-fibers) are stimulated, the inhibitory interneurons stop firing, which produces an "open gate" situation. This open-gate condition allows incoming pain information to synapse into the ascending, secondary pain fibers and eventually reach higher neural centers (e.g., the thalamus and cerebral cortex), where it is "perceived" as pain (Melzack, 1973).

Supporting the gate control theory is the well-known fact that a contra-irritant, like rubbing one's big toe after stubbing it, does apparently stimulate the larger sensory fibers in the skin and block pain transmission at the spinal level. Still, the theory is unable to account for other findings of recent research concerning "opiate-like" substances that are released by the body during tactile stimulation.

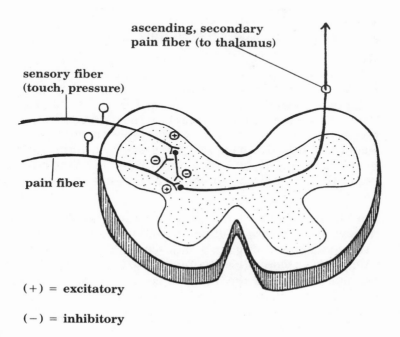

(+) = **excitatory**

(−) = **inhibitory**

FIGURE 21 — **Gate control theory of pain.** A small-diameter sensory nerve (C-fiber) is shown carrying pain information from the periphery to an ascending, secondary pain fiber in the spinal cord. When a large sensory nerve is stimulated (e.g., rubbing, etc.), it blocks or "gates" this pain pathway indirectly through an inhibitory interneuron.

The Endogenous Opiate Theory:
The Endorphins and Enkephalins

With the recent discovery of endogenous peptides (i.e., small proteins made by the body) that bind to opiate receptors in the brain and spinal cord, an "intrinsic analgesic system" has been proposed (Hughes, et al., 1975). This system may help explain the pain-relieving properties of tactile intervention. A number of endogenous opiate peptides have now been isolated: **beta endorphin** (meaning, "the morphine within") and the **enkephalins** (meaning, "in the head") being the most notable.

Initial investigations indicated that the analgesic actions of acupuncture treatments can be reversed by the opiate receptor antagonist, naloxone (Pomeranz and Chiu, 1976). More recently, "electro-acupuncture" administered to mice produced a decrease in naloxone-precipitated "opiate withdrawal," suggesting that the electrical stimulation increased the levels of beta endorphin in neural tissue (Ho, et al., 1978).

Direct measurements of the endogenous opiate levels have also been conducted. Electro-acupuncture increased peripheral circulating levels of beta-endorphin in human subjects (Malizia, et al., 1979). An increase in beta-endorphin levels in cerebrospinal fluid levels following acupuncture therapy has also been reported (Sjolund, Terenius, and Eriksson, 1977).

The exact method by which tactile pressure, needles, and electrical current activate the endogenous opiate system is not fully understood. However, two theoretical models have been put forth: the "neurotransmitter" model and the "hormone" model.

One model emphasizes the role of enkephalins as a "neurotransmitter substance" which is released at synaptic junctions between neurons within the central system itself (Lewis, et al., 1981; Weyhenmeyer, 1983). This so-called "hardwire" theory proposes that sensory stimulation (e.g., somato-procedures) directly excites neural circuits in the brain and spinal cord, causing the release of the peptide opiates.

It is known, for example, that stimulation of certain brain centers (i.e., parts of the thalamus and brainstem) induced a general analgesia (Lewis, et al., 1981).

The neural "hardwire" circuitry or pathway may be outlined as follows:

1. Certain incoming sensory information (e.g., tactile pressure) eventually synapses in the thalamus and brainstem.
2. Neurons from these regions project to another area in the brainstem (i.e., the **Raphe nuclei**).
3. The Raphe nuclei in turn send neurons that terminate on interneurons in the spinal cord.
4. These interneurons then release enkephalins that inhibit ascending secondary pain fibers. (See Figure 22.)

The second model describes the opiate peptides as "hormone-like" in their actions. Specifically, the pituitary gland releases beta endorphins into the circulating blood, which transports them to their target organs, the brain and spinal cord. In the spinal cord, the endorphins block pain transmission to higher centers (Henry, 1982).

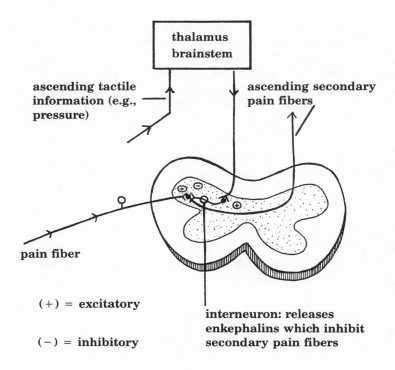

FIGURE 22 — **Enkephalins as a neurotransmitter:** (1) incoming tactile information is sent to the thalamus and brainstem; (2) from the brainstem (Raphe nuclei), a neuron carries output to an interneuron in the spinal cord; and (3) this interneuron releases enkephalins as a neurotransmitter that in turn inhibits pain information from traveling up an ascending secondary pain fiber.

The actual pathway and mechanism of the hormone model may be stated as follows:

1. Tactile sensory information is sent to the higher neural centers including the **hypothalamus.**
2. Impulses from the hypothalamus project to the **pituitary gland** of the endocrine system.
3. The pituitary releases beta endorphins into general circulation.
4. The circulating endorphins then pass through the "blood brain barrier" into the brain and spinal cord.
5. In the spinal cord, the beta endorphins block the transmission of pain at the synapses of incoming sensory fibers.

The fact that acupuncture analgesia is reduced by removal of the pituitary gland supports the "hormone" model position that the pituitary secretes beta endorphins into the blood stream (Pomeranz, Cheng, and Law, 1977).

The endorphins and enkephalins appear to be concerned with more than regulating pain. It has been speculated that through the nervous system, they have global effects on autonomic function (e.g., heart rate, blood pressure, and respiration) as well as on social behaviors (Henry, 1982).

In conclusion, the "neurotransmitter" and the "hormone" models are not mutually exclusive. Both describe mechanisms by which tactile intervention evokes the release of the analgesic peptides. Perhaps "neuro-hormone" is the most appropriate term for these substances.

Therapeutic Benefits

For thousands of years, man has applied massage, deep pressure, and needles to specific points on the skin's surface for the relief of pain.

Recent experimental investigations have uncovered mechanisms that partially explain how these techniques obtain their often remarkable results. Though neither the gate control theory or the two endogenous opiate models completely account for the analgesic effects, they have given somato-therapies credibility as treatments for a wide scope of pain-related problems as well as for anesthetic purposes.

Somato-techniques are currently utilized in pain management for the following conditions:

1. Soft-tissue pain in the neck, shoulders, back, knees, etc. (also see Chapter 13)
2. Pain that is related to various "neuralgias" (i.e., irritation of nerve tissue)
3. Osteoarthritic pain found in joints
4. The pain of muscular and migraine headaches

REFERENCES

Becker, R.O., et al. Electrophysiological correlates of acupuncture points and meridians. *Psychoenergetic Systems,* 1976, *1* 105–112.

Chu, L., Yeh, S., and Wood, D. *Acupuncture Manual: a Western Approach.* New York: M. Dekker, 1979.

Henry, F.L. Circulating opioids: possible physiological roles in central nervous function. *Neuroscience and Biobehavioral Reviews,* 1982, *6,* 229–245.

Ho, W.K.K., et al. The influence of electroacupuncture on naloxone-induced morphine withdrawal in mice: elevation of brain opiate activity. *Eur. J. Pharmac.,* 1978, *49,* 197–199.

Hughes, J., et al. Purification and properties of enkephalin—the possible endogenous ligand for the morphine receptor. *Life Science,* 1975, *16,* 1753–1758.

Lewis, J.W., et al. Possible role of opioid peptides in pain inhibition and seizures. In J.B. Martin, S. Reichlin, K.L. Bick (Eds.), *Advances in Biochemical Psychopharmacology* (Vol. 28). New York: Raven Press, 1981.

Malizia, E., et al. Electroacupuncture and peripheral beta-endorphin and ACTH levels. *Lancet,* 1979, *2,* 535.

Melzack, R. How acupuncture can block pain. *Impact of Science on Society,* 1973, *23,* 65–75.

Melzack, R., Stillwell, D.M., and Fox, E.J. Trigger points and acupuncture points for pain: correlations and implications. *PAIN,* 1977, *3,* 3–23.

Oschman, J.L. *The Connective Tissue and Myofascial Systems.* Berkeley, CA: Aspen Research Institute, 1981.

Pomeranz, B., and Chiu, D. Naloxone blockade of acupuncture analgesia: endorphin implicated. *Life Science,* 1976, *19,* 1757–1762.

Pomeranz, B., Cheng, R., and Law, P. Acupuncture reduces electrophysiological and behavioral responses to noxious stimuli: pituitary is implicated. *Expl. Neural.,* 1977, *54,* 172–178.

Sjolund, R., Terenius, L., and Eriksson, M. Increased cerebrospinal fluid levels of endorphins after electro-acupuncture. *Acta Physiologica Scandinavica,* 1977, *100,* 382–384.

Weyhenmeyer, J. Fall, 1983. Lectures in Functional Neuroanatomy 407 at the University of Illinois, (Urbana-Champaign).

... A fuller understanding of life will be achieved only by developing a "systems biology," a biology that sees an organism as a living system rather than a machine.

— *Fritjof Capra*

CHAPTER 19
PHYSIOLOGICAL EVIDENCE: CONCLUSIONS

> There are more things in heaven and earth, Horatio,
> than are dreamt of in your philosophy.
>
> —Hamlet
> *W. Shakespeare*

The effects of somato-procedures on physiological function is a field of inquiry that is largely uncharted. Still, some definite inferences can be made. The physiological consequences of touch-oriented interventions may be placed in two broad domains:

1. **Direct local responses** in the tissues under stimulation
2. **Indirect global responses** regulated by the nervous system and possibly the connective-tissue network

The first domain would include the mechanical effects of stroking and pressure on the arterial, venous, and lymphatic movements as well as the relief of pain caused by restricted (i.e., ischemic) circulation.

There is also evidence that deep pressure and compression to the fascial connective tissue cause temporary changes in its ground substance (from a semisolid to a liquid-like condition), thus allowing alterations of its shape and thickness. Connective tissue's attribute of "plasticity" has significant implications for the body's musculoskeletal structure.

The second domain of effects involves systemic physiological responses mediated and regulated through the nervous system.

Various types of somato-procedures have been demonstrated to change neuromuscular functions including muscle tone, posture, and complex movement.

Similarly, autonomic functions are affected by various "vagotonic" and "sympathicotonic" manipulations. This tactile stimulation of the sensory or afferent pathways elicits autonomic reflexes and may have profound implications for long-term autonomic functioning as well.

Tactile methods are also known to induce systemic effects on the perception of pain. Levels of the endogenous opiate peptides—the endorphins and enkephalins—increase after certain somato-procedures. These "neuro-hormones" block or inhibit the transmission of pain information from the spinal cord to higher brain centers.

Finally, fascia and other types of connective tissue appear to act as "semiconductors," permitting the movement of electrical charge through the fascial web. Correlations have been made between the "meridians" of traditional acupuncture theory and the fascial planes of the body. Thus, the connective tissue may form an electrical circuit of its own—a second communication network that complements the nervous system.

The known and potential therapeutic benefits of body therapies are impressive. There is reason to infer, from both case reports and experimental investigations, that somato-techniques are appropriate treatments for:

1. Muscle spasms common in athletic injuries
2. General stress management

3. Neuromuscular and neurological disorders including cerebral palsy, stroke, and coma
4. Postural and movement-related problems
5. Chronic pain syndromes such as headaches, joint pain, and neuralgias

The consequences of touch on the body's "subsystems" (circulatory, connective tissue, nervous, etc.) have been presented chapter by chapter as if the effects were separate and distinct for each subsystem. Such an approach of examining the human being as a group of discrete, physiological parts has limitations, particularly for understanding the global, integrating role of somato-interventions.

However, a new perspective is gaining recognition in the biological sciences based on "general systems theory" (Capra, 1982; Garfinkel, 1984). From a systems-theory viewpoint, the functional physiological variables, or subsystems of the body, are seen as a dynamic interrelated whole.

Garfinkel (1984) has recently proposed that the body's subsystems are not involved in merely maintaining a steady state of equilibrium or "homeostasis," as has long been assumed. Rather, the subsystems appear to "oscillate" through "regular high-low cycles"; and a harmony or synchronization along the oscillating subsystems (i.e., a "phase coherence") seems to exist.

To truly understand somato-procedures' physiological consequences, the rhythmic patterns of these physiological variables must be explored. Indeed, a "physiological integration of action" concerning the body's subsystems may become the model of future biological investigations (Adolf, 1982).

Like the limitations of Horatio's "philosophy," there are "more things" in physiology than classical biological theory ever imagined.

REFERENCES

Adolf, E. Physiological integrations in action. *Physiologist,* 1982, *25*(2), (April).

Garfinkel, A. Attractors and stages of scientific thought. *American Journal of Physiology,* 1984, *245,* 455–566.

Capra, F. *The Turning Point.* New York: Simon and Schuster, 1982.

INDEX

Acupuncture, 1-10, 13, 39, 44, 56, 84, 89, 108, 121, 124, 165, 168, 171, 172, 178

Alexander, F.M., 59-63, 71

Alexander technique, 59-63, 67, 71, 89, 137, 138, 139, 140, 141-142

Alignment, 59, 68, 71, 134

Alpha motor neuron, 130-136

Anesthesia, 10, 172

Applied kinesiology, 56

Arthritis, 172

Asanas, 13, 70

Asclepiades, 27-28

Asthma, 54, 62, 159, 160

Athletic injuries, 141, 142, 178
muscle cramps, 141

Autonomic balance, 9, 147-162
diseases and disorders, 159-160
flexibility, 152, 155-160
law of reciprocal innervation, 155
autonomic rebound, 150, 157, 160
autonomic tuning, 150, 159-160

Autonomic nervous system, 9, 20, 69-70, 77-78, 118, 120, 136, 147-151, 171, 178

Autonomic reflexes, 151-155, 178
depressor reflex, 153
pressor reflex, 154

somato-procedures' effects, 154-155

Ayurvedic medicine, 14, 19-21

Back pain, 54, 124, 172

Bartenieff, I., 86

Basic movement, 85-86

Body image, 84

Bonesetters, 32

Bioenergetics, 79

Brain
basal ganglia, 119-120, 134-135
brainstem, 117, 134-135, 147, 169, 170
cerebellum, 119-120, 134-135
cerebral cortex, 119-120, 134-135, 138, 166
hypothalamus, 119-120, 147, 153, 171
limbic system, 119-120, 147, 153
subcortical structures, 119, 139, 140
thalamus, 119-120, 134-135, 166, 169, 170

Breathing, 13, 76

Caduceus, 15-16

Central nervous system, 20, 46, 117-118, 121-123, 168-171

Index

Tonification-sedation, 7, 56
Touch for Health, 10, 56
Trigger points, 165

Vagal tone, 154, 155-158
Vedic scriptures, 13, 19, 20
Venous flow, 38, 96

Whiplash, 124

Yin-yang, 1-10, 15, 79,
150-151

THE AUTHOR

John T. Cottingham is a practitioner of the Rolfing method of soft-tissue manipulation, working both in private practice and at the Frances Nelson Health Center in Champaign, Illinois. He has recently received his Master's degree in the biological sciences from the University of Illinois and is involved in research concerning manipulative therapy and the autonomic nervous system. John has lectured and conducted workshops on body therapies at the Rolf Institute, University of Illinois, and Parkland College. He is currently designing a semester course in somatotechniques for health-care students at Parkland College. John lives with his wife, Mary Rose, in Urbana, Illinois.